THE VAGUS NERVE SOLUTION

OPTIMIZE TOTAL BODY HEALTH WITH SIMPLE
TECHNIQUES TO REDUCE STRESS, SOOTHE
ANXIETY, IMPROVE DIGESTION, AND EASE
CHRONIC PAIN

LORILEE LUCAS

Published in the United States by Everwell Publishing 2024

No part of this publication may be reproduced in any form without written permission from the publisher.

Paperback ISBN: 978-1-965625-03-3
Hardback ISBN: 978-1-965625-02-6
Ebook ISBN: 978-1-965625-01-9

Book Cover Design by Darko Bovan
Internal Illustrations by Aya Suarjaya

For permissions, bulk orders, or speaking engagements, email:
everwellpublishing@gmail.com

To the weary souls seeking answers,

May you find the healing, peace, and vitality you deserve.

This book is for you.

CONTENTS

EMBARK ON YOUR VAGUS NERVE ADVENTURE

The vagus nerve might sound like just another scientific term, but for me, it has been a lifeline—one that has played a pivotal role in my own healing journey. After a near-death experience in 2007, I embarked on a path to rebuild my body and spirit with an unwavering commitment to self-care. Years later, when a cascade of losses presented new challenges—losing my home and belongings in a wildfire, losing my career and financial stability to the global pandemic, and enduring the heart-wrenching end of a long-term marriage, all while facing a serious health diagnosis—I knew I had to find the strength to reframe these losses as an opportunity so I could rebuild my life.

At the heart of that journey, I discovered the transformative power of the vagus nerve, a biological pathway that connects so many of our body's vital systems. By learning how to tap into this internal network, I was able to regain control of my life in ways I never thought possible. This book is the culmination of that journey and the scientific research I relied on to support my path to wellness.

You might be facing similar challenges—persistent stress, anxiety, or chronic pain—and you're looking for answers. Whether it's digestive issues, brain fog, or the weight of unresolved trauma, it can feel overwhelming. I understand because I've been there. But the good news is that your body already holds the key to healing. The vagus nerve is your body's built-in healing mechanism; once you learn how to engage it, the transformation can be profound.

In the pages ahead, I'll share not only the science but also practical tools you can use to activate your vagus nerve, regain balance, and begin your healing journey. Together, we'll explore how you can take simple, daily steps to reduce stress, improve digestion, ease chronic pain, and restore vitality.

PART I: UNDERSTANDING THE VAGUS NERVE

STRUCTURE AND FUNCTION

CHAPTER 1
ANATOMY AND PHYSIOLOGY OF THE VAGUS NERVE

A JOURNEY INSIDE

The vagus nerve is finally having its moment in the spotlight, and for good reason. Did you know this unsung hero is responsible for the invisible yet crucial dialogue between your brain and several vital organs - quietly playing a monumental role in your body's daily functions? This conversation, facilitated by the vagus nerve, underpins everything from your gut feelings to how calmly you can respond to stress. It's high time for the vagus nerve to take center stage so we can all begin to tap into the power within each of us. Understanding this superstar nerve isn't just academic; it's a step towards gaining control over the unconscious processes that affect your health in profound yet practical ways.

The vagus nerve is known as the "wandering nerve" because of its extensive reach. It touches numerous organs as it travels from the brainstem throughout the body. It begins its journey rooted in the medulla oblongata, a part of the brainstem that serves as a control hub for autonomic functions like breathing and heart rate. From there, it descends, branching out intricately and bilaterally from the neck to the chest and abdomen.

As you trace its path, imagine the vagus nerve as a major highway that exits the brainstem, then splits and meanders to various critical stops—your heart, lungs, liver, spleen, pancreas, and intestines. Each branch of this nerve carries bundles of fibers tasked with specific roles, delivering messages that adjust the function of these organs. For instance, the branches that interface with your heart regulate heartbeat speed, ensuring that it beats slower during moments of calm and faster when you need more oxygen during activities.

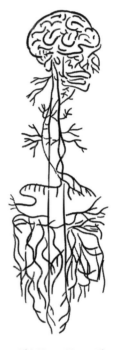

The Vagus Nerve: The tenth cranial nerve, connecting the brain to several organ structures

At its core, the vagus nerve comprises many branches containing sensory and motor fibers. These fibers are the communication lines; sensory fibers gather information from the organs, sending it back to the brain and providing updates on the state of internal affairs. Motor fibers, conversely, carry messages from the brain to the organs. This bi-directional communication is crucial for maintaining homeostasis, the body's way of keeping its internal environment stable and balanced despite external changes.

A closer look at these fibers reveals their importance in bodily functions. The nerve consists mainly of two types of fibers. Afferent fibers, making up about 80% of the nerve, send sensory signals from the body to the brain. These signals inform the brain about various conditions, such as the presence of food in the gut or states of inflammation or relaxation. Though fewer in number, efferent fibers are crucial for sending motor commands from the brain to the organs. These fibers regulate essential processes like digestion by controlling acid secretion in the stomach and enzyme production in the pancreas.

Interestingly, the vagus nerve operates bilaterally but not symmetrically, meaning that while it runs on both the left and right sides of your body, they perform slightly different functions due to their path and organ connections. For example, the right vagus nerve tends to have more influence over the heart, helping to reduce heart rate. In contrast, the left has more extensive branches to the digestive tract, influencing gastrointestinal functions. This asymmetrical control allows the body to manage its resources effectively, responding adaptively to various physiological demands.

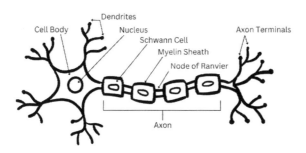

Anatomy of a Neuron

The protective and insulating layers around nerve fibers are called myelin sheaths. This myelination process speeds up electrical signal transmission along the nerve. The degree of myelination in the vagus nerve impacts how quickly and efficiently messages are communicated between the brain and the body. Highly myelinated fibers transmit signals swiftly, allowing for rapid responses to environmental changes, which is vital for functions that need immediate action, such as heart rate regulation during stressful situations.

CHAPTER 2

VAGUS NERVE IN HEALTH AND DISEASE
THE SILENT INFLUENCER

I magine a symphony where each instrument is perfectly tuned to create a harmonious and moving performance. Now, think of your body as that orchestra and the vagus nerve as the conductor, with its tone influencing the overall health and balance of your body's systems. Just as the conductor's baton guides the flow and intensity of the music, so too does the vagus nerve guide the intricate interactions within your body. This chapter delves into the concept of vagal tone— what it is, why it matters, and how you can enhance it to conduct a healthier, more resilient life.

VAGAL TONE EXPLAINED: WHY IT MATTERS FOR YOUR HEALTH

Vagal tone refers to the activity level of your vagus nerve. Measured primarily through heart rate variability (HRV), vagal tone offers a window into your body's ability to manage stress and maintain internal balance. High HRV indicates a healthy, responsive vagus nerve that can effectively regulate your body's systems, promoting relaxation and recovery.

Conversely, low HRV is often a sign of stress, where the body struggles to shift smoothly from states of arousal to relaxation, potentially leading to various health issues.

The measurement of HRV involves analyzing the time variation between consecutive heartbeats, which should naturally vary as you breathe in and out. During inhalation, your heart rate typically speeds up slightly, and during exhalation, it slows down. The vagus nerve orchestrates this subtle dance between your heart rate and breathing and is a critical indicator of your overall health and resilience.

Why should you care about vagal tone? Because it's an excellent biomarker for your overall health and your body's resilience against potential diseases. People with higher vagal tone generally have better control over their heart rate, digestion, and emotional responses, making them more capable of coping with stress. A higher vagal tone doesn't just mean they feel calmer; it translates into tangible health benefits, such as lower risk of heart disease, reduced incidence of stroke, better glucose control, and less susceptibility to harmful effects of stress like inflammation.

Moreover, enhancing your vagal tone can be particularly beneficial if you're dealing with chronic conditions such as anxiety, depression, or digestive disorders. It acts almost like a reset button, helping to restore balance to your nervous system and improve your body's ability to heal and maintain optimal function. We will explore methods to stimulate and enhance vagal tone in Part 4 (Chapters 11-19).

POLYVAGAL THEORY: A NEW UNDERSTANDING OF SAFETY AND THREAT

In your quest to understand the vagus nerve, it's essential to explore one of the most influential theories that have reshaped our understanding of how the nervous system influences our responses to stress and safety: Stephen Porges's Polyvagal Theory. This theory offers a fresh perspective on how the nervous system interacts with environmental stimuli to regulate emotional and physiological states. It's particularly revelatory in explaining why and how we react to stress, danger, and social interactions.

Polyvagal Theory breaks down the autonomic nervous system, which controls involuntary body functions, into three distinct neural circuits. It posits that our evolutionary history has resulted in the development of these three circuits, each responsible for different behavioral and physiological responses. The oldest of these is the reptilian system, which governs the primitive freeze response—think of a deer caught in headlights, immobilized by fear. This system is activated when there's a perception of life-threatening danger and no apparent escape route.

Moving up the evolutionary ladder to the mammalian system, we find the sympathetic nervous system, which controls the well-known fight-or-flight response. This system kicks into gear when you perceive a threat you believe you need to overcome or escape from by confrontation or evasion. It primes your body for action, diverting blood to muscles, increasing heart rate, and pumping adrenaline.

According to Polyvagal Theory, the most evolved system is the social engagement system, regulated by the myelinated branches of the vagus nerve. This system is unique to mammals and relies on non-verbal cues such as facial expression and vocal tone to communicate safety and foster positive social interactions. When this system is active, it inhibits the lower, more primitive systems, reducing heart rate and cultivating calm and connectivity. In this way, the vagus nerve truly shines, illustrating its crucial role in modulating our responses to the world around us.

These systems do not operate in isolation. Their hierarchical arrangement allows more evolved systems to inhibit more primitive ones, helping to modulate your response to stress and perceived threats. For instance, a supportive social environment can activate the social engagement system, dampening the fight-or-flight response and promoting feelings of calm. This helps to illuminate why social support is not just comforting but is physiologically soothing and can be a powerful tool in managing stress and recovering from trauma.

The implications of Polyvagal Theory extend deeply into therapeutic settings, especially in treating conditions rooted in traumatic experiences, such as PTSD, anxiety disorders, and various phobias. Therapists can tailor interventions to target these systems by understanding how different triggers activate these neural circuits. For example, therapies that enhance social engagement—such as music, rhythmic movements, and deep listening—can help reactivate the body's natural state of calm and safety.

Moreover, interventions that stimulate the vagus nerve, such as controlled breathing techniques and vagal nerve stimulators, can directly influence these neural circuits. They help shift the body's physiological state from hyperarousal or shutdown (characteristic of the reptilian and mammalian systems) to social engagement and calm. The myelinated vagus nerve mediates this process.

Understanding Polyvagal Theory enriches your comprehension of the vagus nerve's pivotal role in your emotional and physical health. It provides a framework for why certain therapeutic practices are successful and how to apply these insights to manage stress better, build safer social environments, and foster a more resilient nervous system.

As we close this chapter, reflect on how the vagus nerve, through the lens of Polyvagal Theory, plays a fundamental role in navigating the complexities of human behavior and health. This theory reshapes our perspective on stress responses and social interactions while equipping us with practical tools to foster safety and calm. In the next chapter, we will explore specific neurotransmitters influenced by the vagus nerve, deepening your understanding of how this nerve impacts your mental and physical health on a biochemical level.

CHAPTER 3

NEUROTRANSMITTERS AND THE VAGUS NERVE
THE COMMUNICATION HIGHWAY

I magine your body as a bustling city, with the vagus nerve acting as the central communication network, seamlessly connecting different regions to ensure everything runs smoothly. But what are the messages that keep this city thriving? They are neurotransmitters, the body's chemical couriers. Understanding their interaction with the vagus nerve reveals how intricately linked our mental states and physical health truly are. This chapter delves into the vital roles these neurotransmitters play, transmitted through the vagus nerve, influencing everything from your heart rate to your feelings of happiness or anxiety.

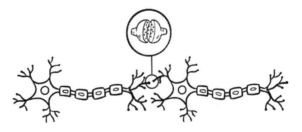

Two Neurons Communicating with Each Other via Neurotransmitters at a Synapse

NEUROTRANSMITTERS AND THE VAGUS NERVE: THE CHEMICAL MESSENGERS

Acetylcholine supervises this communication process, ensuring smooth operations. Primarily released by the vagus nerve, this neurotransmitter is a key player in managing how your heart beats and food digests. When released, it tells your heart to take a beat, quite literally slowing it down during restful periods, promoting calm, and allowing your body to conserve energy. It also oversees the digestive process by signaling the stomach to ramp up the production of digestive acids, helping break down your meals more effectively. This type of regulation is vital for maintaining equilibrium within your body, ensuring that everything is managed efficiently, from nutrient absorption to heart health.

The relationship between your body and brain is not a one-way street; it's a dynamic, two-way communication super-highway with the vagus nerve at its core. This nerve sends sensory information from the body up to the brain, detailing everything from gut discomfort to the sensation of a calm heartbeat. Conversely, it transmits motor commands from the brain back to the body, ensuring that appropriate actions ensue to maintain homeostasis—a stable, balanced internal environment. For instance, if you're facing a stressor, the brain uses the vagus nerve to tell your heart to beat faster, preparing you to handle the situation. This bidirectional flow of information is crucial for your body to adapt swiftly and effectively to internal and external changes.

The vagus nerve also plays a pivotal role in regulating mood and stress levels, interfacing closely with neurotransmitters like serotonin and GABA (gamma-aminobutyric acid). Serotonin, often dubbed the 'feel-good' neurotransmitter, influences various functions, from mood and emotions to sleep and appetite. The vagus nerve helps regulate serotonin levels, enhancing your mood and promoting a sense of well-being. GABA, the primary inhibitory neurotransmitter in the brain, works to reduce neuronal excitability throughout the nervous system. Through its action, the vagus nerve can influence GABA levels, helping to calm the brain and reduce feelings of anxiety and stress. This modulation of neurotransmitters by the vagus nerve is why it's sometimes possible to 'breathe through' a stressful moment or why you might feel calmer after vagus-stimulating exercises.

Research has increasingly shown the close link between vagal activity and mental health conditions, including depression and anxiety. Low vagal tone correlates with increased stress responses and mood imbalances. By understanding how to stimulate the vagus nerve, you can directly enhance its tone, which can help elevate levels of beneficial neurotransmitters and lower the stress-reactive chemicals in your brain. This approach offers promising avenues for not only understanding but also treating various mental health conditions by natural and non-invasive means.

Beyond its psychological impacts, the vagus nerve influences physical aspects of health, such as digestive processes and immune response. It helps manage inflammation, a common culprit behind myriad health issues, through a pathway known as the 'cholinergic anti-inflammatory pathway.' By releasing acetylcholine, the vagus nerve can inhibit the production of cytokines, which are proteins involved in inflammation. This mechanism is crucial in managing conditions like irritable bowel syndrome (IBS), where inflammation plays a significant role. Moreover, this anti-inflammatory effect is not just limited to the gut; it extends to other areas of the body, offering potential relief from autoimmune diseases and arthritis.

Another area of keen interest is the vagus nerve's role in modulating pain. Through its anti-inflammatory actions, the vagus nerve can also influence how pain is perceived and managed. By reducing the underlying inflammation, the nerve can help alleviate the sensation of pain. This connection is particularly relevant for chronic pain conditions, where inflammation often exacerbates the pain experience. Understanding and harnessing this function of the vagus nerve opens up new pathways for managing chronic pain, potentially reducing reliance on medications and improving quality of life.

The interplay between neurotransmitters and the vagus nerve reveals the connections between mental and physical health. By fine-tuning this dance through techniques that enhance vagal tone, you can soothe your mind and heal your body.

NEUROTRANSMITTER IMBALANCES

Neurotransmitters play a pivotal role in the intricate dance of your body's internal communications. They are the chemicals your brain cells use to tell your heart to beat, your lungs to breathe, and your stomach to digest. However, like anything in life, balance is essential, and imbalances in these crucial chemicals can lead to a cascade of health issues, impacting everything from your mood to your physical health.

One of the most common neurotransmitter imbalances involves serotonin, often called the "feel-good" neurotransmitter. Serotonin helps regulate mood, appetite, and sleep, among other things. Because serotonin contributes to feelings of well-being, when levels fall, it can lead to feelings of depression and anxiety. Low levels can remove this buffer against the small stresses of everyday life, making you feel more susceptible to anxiety and depressive states.

Dopamine is another crucial player in the realm of neurotransmitters, often dubbed the "reward" chemical because it is released whenever we do something pleasurable. It's vital for motivation, pleasure, and reward. Low dopamine levels can result in a lack of motivation, fatigue, addictive behavior, mood swings, and memory loss. On the flip side, an excess of dopamine is linked to hyperactivity and impulsivity, as seen in conditions like ADHD.

Another vital neurotransmitter is GABA (gamma-aminobutyric acid), which primarily acts as an inhibitor in the brain, meaning it blocks specific brain signals and decreases activity in the nervous system. When GABA levels are too low, it can lead to anxiety, chronic stress, and even conditions like epilepsy. In contrast, too much GABA can lead to sedation and a decrease in motor and cognitive capabilities, which might manifest as excessive fatigue or lethargy.

The symptoms of neurotransmitter imbalances can vary widely depending on which chemical is out of balance and whether it is in excess or deficit. Common signs include mood swings, anxiety, depression, sleep problems, fatigue, weight issues, and observable changes in appetite or sex drive. These symptoms can often be subtle and increase in intensity over time, making them easy to overlook until they become more severe.

Often, diagnosing these imbalances involves a combination of symptom assessment, medical history, and, sometimes, specialized tests that can measure levels of specific neuro-transmitters in your blood or urine. Treatment options range from dietary changes, lifestyle modifications, and supplements to therapies aimed at balancing neurotransmitter levels.

Understanding and addressing neurotransmitter imbalances is crucial for managing overall health. By recognizing symptoms and exploring treatment options, you can take proactive steps towards better mental and physical well-being.

Neurotransmitters play a vital role in the complex communication network within your body, significantly influencing your mental and physical health. By maintaining balance in these chemical messengers through lifestyle choices and therapeutic interventions, you can enhance your overall well-being. In the next chapter, we'll examine how these imbalances can be diagnosed and effectively managed, continuing our exploration into neurotransmitters' critical role in our overall well-being.

PART II: NAVIGATING HEALTH AND SAFETY WITH THE VAGUS NERVE

CHAPTER 4

DIAGNOSTICS AND TESTING
GETTING TO THE ROOT

I magine stepping into a secret mission where decoding your body's subtle signals can unlock the ultimate health secrets. In this chapter, we explore the diagnostics and testing of the vagus nerve, a critical yet often overlooked component of our nervous system. Why focus on this one nerve? Think of the vagus nerve as the secret agent of your body, quietly influencing your emotional balance, heart function, digestion, and overall resilience with stealth. Learning to assess and enhance its function allows you to harness this agent's power, setting the stage for a healthier, more vibrant life.

ASSESSING VAGAL TONE: KEY INDICATORS

The first step in harnessing the healing power of the vagus nerve is to understand its current state of activity, often referred to as vagal tone. Two primary physiological markers provide insight into this hidden world: respiratory sinus arrhythmia (RSA) and heart rate variability (HRV). These indicators are crucial as they reflect how well your vagus nerve regulates heart rate changes during breathing cycles—essentially, how quickly your body can relax after experiencing stress.

RSA is a phenomenon where your heart rate speeds up during inhalation and slows down during exhalation. This natural ebb and flow indicates a flexible and healthy vagus nerve. On the other hand, HRV is the variation in time between each heartbeat, directly influenced by your autonomic nervous system—the system that controls bodily functions not consciously directed, such as breathing, the heartbeat, and digestive processes. A higher HRV suggests a robust vagal tone, indicating an effective and resilient stress-response system.

Understanding your baseline measurements for these indicators is akin to knowing the starting point on a map before embarking on a journey. It's about understanding where you are to chart where you need to go. Establishing these markers helps to track the progress of interventions—whether they're lifestyle changes, therapies, or exercises designed to improve vagal tone. Regular monitoring allows you to see the immediate effects of a single change and the long-term trends that inform whether the interventions are working.

So, how are these measurements taken? Thankfully, with technological advances, assessing your vagal tone is becoming easier and more accessible. Devices such as smartwatches and ECG monitors can now measure HRV in real-time, providing immediate feedback about your body's stress levels and autonomic function. These devices use sensors to detect heartbeats and calculate the variability between them, offering insights into how well your vagus nerve is functioning. Whether done in clinical settings by healthcare professionals or at home with consumer-grade devices, it allows for continuous monitoring without invasive procedures.

Recognizing that several external factors can influence vagal tone readings is crucial. Stress, sleep quality, physical fitness, and even your hydration levels can alter HRV and RSA. For instance, a poor night's sleep or high stress can temporarily lower HRV, reflecting a strain on your body's resources. Similarly, regular physical activity can improve HRV over time, indicating enhanced vagal tone and a more resilient stress response system. Understanding these factors provides a more holistic view of your health. It helps tailor interventions more effectively, ensuring they address the symptoms and root causes affecting your vagal health.

By taking the time to understand and measure your vagal tone, you're taking an essential step in tuning into your body's unique rhythms and needs. This chapter gives you the knowledge to interpret these vital signs and empowers you to make informed decisions about your health interventions. As we move forward, remember that each piece of data is a stepping stone towards a deeper understanding of your body and a healthier, more balanced life.

HEART RATE VARIABILITY AND VAGUS NERVE HEALTH

When you think about your heart's rhythms, you might picture it beating steadily like a drum, maintaining a consistent tempo. Yet, the reality is that it is far more nuanced and dynamic. Heart Rate Variability (HRV) measures these subtle variations in the time between each heartbeat, far from random noise; they provide critical insights into your autonomic nervous system's health and balance. This variability echoes your body's ability to adapt to stress, recover from exertion, and handle life's challenges.

HRV is influenced directly by the vagus nerve, which acts as a brake when your heart rate speeds up due to stress or physical demands. A higher HRV indicates a strong vagal tone, meaning your body can effectively slow down the heart rate and promote relaxation faster following stress. How well you can switch from a state of alert (fight or flight) to a state of rest (rest and digest) is fundamental to maintaining overall health and resilience.

The relationship between HRV and various health outcomes is profound. For instance, higher HRV indicates better cardiovascular health, lower stress levels, and increased resilience to physical and psychological stressors. Conversely, a lower HRV correlates with conditions such as anxiety, depression, heart disease, and increased risk of sudden cardiac death. It's not just about how fast your heart beats but how well your heart adjusts its pace to suit your body's needs.

Improving your HRV and, by extension, your vagal tone can have far-reaching benefits for your health. Effective methods to enhance HRV include meditation, which helps regulate the body's stress response by promoting relaxation and mindfulness. Regular aerobic exercise is another powerful tool. Improving heart efficiency and lung capacity enhances overall cardiovascular health, thereby improving HRV. Additionally, simple breathing techniques, such as slow, deep breathing, can stimulate the vagus nerve directly, slowing down the heart rate and increasing HRV.

To bring these points home, consider the findings from various studies that demonstrate the impact of these interventions on HRV. Research has shown that individuals who engage in regular meditation or yoga can significantly increase their HRV over time, reflecting enhanced autonomic control and decreased stress levels. Aerobic exercise has similar effects, with studies indicating that routine physical activity can lead to long-term improvements in HRV, suggesting a more resilient cardiovascular system.

These insights underscore HRV's value as a marker of current health and a predictor of future well-being, offering a roadmap for interventions that can profoundly impact your quality of life. By understanding and applying techniques to improve HRV, you are taking proactive steps toward enhancing your vagal health, equipping your body to manage stress better, and paving the way for a healthier, more balanced existence.

BIOFEEDBACK: LISTENING TO YOUR BODY'S SIGNALS

In your pursuit of understanding and enhancing the function of your vagus nerve, one of the most empowering tools at your disposal is biofeedback. This technology might sound futuristic, but it's rooted in a simple principle. By monitoring your physiological processes, you can learn to control them more effectively, turning involuntary bodily responses into conscious actions. Biofeedback harnesses the signals from your body, such as heart rate or muscle tension, and feeds this information back to you in real-time. This feedback can be crucial in teaching you how to make subtle changes in your body to alleviate symptoms of stress, anxiety, and pain.

At its core, biofeedback is about gaining more control over your physiological states. For instance, by observing how your heart rate varies with breathing, you can learn to control your breath to maximize heart rate variability (HRV). This kind of self-regulation doesn't just help in managing stress; it can also be instrumental in addressing issues like hypertension, chronic pain, and anxiety.

Biofeedback devices use sensors to measure physiological parameters such as heart rate, skin conductivity, muscle tension, and brainwave patterns. The data is collected and translated into a readable format, often displayed on a screen or through audio cues, enabling you to observe how your body reacts to stress, relaxation, or intentional adjustments.

The core advantage of biofeedback is real-time feedback, allowing you to experiment with different methods to consciously regulate your body's responses. For example, slow, deep breathing reduces your heart rate and muscle tension, providing immediate evidence that your actions have a direct physiological impact.

Biofeedback is crucial for fostering behavioral change. Awareness of your body's responses to stress or relaxation techniques helps you develop healthier habits and change harmful behaviors. Regular biofeedback sessions reinforce these behaviors, integrating them into your daily routine. This is especially beneficial for conditions like anxiety, where physiological symptoms can be severe and disruptive.

Biofeedback appears in various health contexts. It effectively manages stress by reinforcing relaxation techniques that reduce physiological stress markers. For those with anxiety, biofeedback sessions can help calm the nervous system, alleviating physical symptoms of anxiety disorders. It can be used in chronic pain management, teaching individuals to relax specific muscles to reduce pain. Additionally, biofeedback can improve heart rate variability (HRV), positively influence vagal tone, and promote better health and resilience.

Examples of Biofeedback Devices

Various biofeedback devices are available, each suited to different needs and health goals.

1. **Heart rate monitors (HRM):** HRMs are the most commonly used and can provide real-time data on heart rate variability. These devices teach users how to control their heart rate through breathing and relaxation techniques.
2. **Electroencephalography (EEG):** EEG devices take a different approach by monitoring brainwave patterns. They are often used in biofeedback to help manage attention disorders and stress-related conditions, providing feedback that helps users learn to produce brainwave patterns associated with calm and focus.
3. **Electromyography (EMG**): EMG devices measure muscle activity. They are handy for reducing muscle tension and managing conditions like back pain or headaches caused by muscle strain.

4. **Heart Rate Variability (HRV) Devices:** Devices, such as "HeartMath," specifically target HRV and coherence to provide feedback designed to improve synchronization between the heart and the brain, enhancing emotional balance and physiological resilience.

5. **Pulse meters**, which are more straightforward in function, measure blood flow and can give insights into how your body responds to stress or relaxation exercises, helping you develop better control over your stress responses.

6. **Respiratory Biofeedback Devices**: These devices monitor breathing patterns and provide feedback to help users develop deeper, slower breathing techniques. These techniques stimulate the vagus nerve and promote relaxation.

7. **Skin Conductance Devices**: These devices measure the skin's electrical conductance, which changes with sweat gland activity in response to stress. By providing feedback on stress levels, they help users practice techniques to reduce stress and enhance vagal tone.

While diverse, these tools all aim to enhance awareness and control over your body's functions, empowering you to manage your health and well-being actively. Through regular use and practice, biofeedback can help you fine-tune your body's responses, significantly improving your physical and mental health and, ultimately, a greater sense of control and quality of life.

In the following sections, we will explore how these technologies are applied and their specific benefits in treating various conditions, further deepening your understanding and ability to harness this powerful tool.

UNLOCKING LAB RESULTS: INSIGHTS INTO THE VAGUS NERVE

When navigating through the complex terrain of your health, understanding the underlying issues can sometimes feel like trying to solve a puzzle without all the pieces. Lab tests provide those missing pieces, offering crucial insights into your body's internal workings, particularly in relation to the vagus nerve. Lab tests can measure everything from inflammation markers to neurotransmitter levels, providing a snapshot of the underlying processes that affect vagal nerve function.

Inflammatory markers, such as C-reactive protein (CRP) or interleukin-6 (IL-6), are vital indicators. Since the vagus nerve regulates inflammation via the cholinergic anti-inflammatory pathway, elevated levels of these markers suggest impaired vagal function. Conversely, a healthy vagus nerve typically correlates with lower systemic inflammation.

Another critical area is the gut microbiome. As part of the gut-brain axis, it has a bidirectional relationship with the vagus nerve. Gut microbiome tests can reveal imbalances that may affect vagal function, contributing to symptoms of anxiety or depression. Restoring balance in gut bacteria most often improves vagal tone and overall well-being.

Neurotransmitter levels in the blood or urine, such as serotonin, dopamine, and GABA, can also indicate how well your vagus nerve functions. Abnormal levels of these neurotransmitters can signal vagal nerve dysfunction, given the nerve's role in regulating these chemicals.

Understanding these results in the context of vagus nerve health requires a nuanced approach. For instance, elevated inflammatory markers that ordinarily suggest issues like infection or chronic inflammation could indicate reduced vagal activity, given its role in inflammation control. Similarly, alterations in gut microbiome profiles could point towards dietary issues, antibiotic use, or vagal nerve dysfunction, requiring different interventions.

Combining lab results with physical assessments like HRV measurements provides a comprehensive view of vagal health, linking biochemical data with physiological responses. For instance, if lab tests show high inflammation but HRV data indicates a strong vagal tone, the issue might be more related to external factors like recent illness or temporary stress rather than chronic vagal dysfunction.

Regular monitoring becomes vital to gather more data and observe patterns. Typically, it's advisable to retest every 3-6 months, depending on the initial findings and the specific interventions you've implemented. More frequent testing might be necessary if the results show significant abnormalities or if you're undergoing treatment for the vagus nerve, such as vagus nerve stimulation therapy.

Consult healthcare professionals specializing in autonomic nervous system disorders for targeted interventions, including lifestyle changes, dietary adjustments, or specific medical treatments. Ensure follow-ups are tailored to your health profile, considering lab results and overall health goals.

By understanding and acting on diagnostic data, you are taking proactive steps toward managing symptoms and treating root causes. These tools guide you toward a balanced, healthy life in which the vagus nerve plays a vital role. In the following sections, we will explore therapeutic techniques to enhance vagal health, providing practical strategies to harness your body's natural healing abilities.

CHAPTER 5

TREATING THE VAGUS NERVE

BALANCING REPAIR, RISKS, AND REWARDS

With its extensive reach, the vagus nerve quietly but powerfully influences your health, touching on everything from how you digest food to how you respond to stress. But what happens when this crucial nerve is compromised? Understanding the causes and consequences of vagus nerve damage and strategies for repair and regeneration can offer hope and practical paths toward healing.

DAMAGE AND REPAIR OF THE VAGUS NERVE

Like any other body part, the vagus nerve can be susceptible to damage. This damage can arise from a variety of sources: physical trauma, surgery, chronic illnesses, or even excessive stress. Each of these sources can disrupt the delicate balance and function of the vagus nerve, leading to a cascade of health issues that might seem unrelated at first glance.

Physical trauma or surgeries near areas where the vagus nerve travels, such as the neck or chest, can inadvertently affect its function. For example, complications from thyroid surgery or car accidents involving significant impact on the neck can lead to direct physical damage. Chronic conditions like diabetes or infections can lead to neuropathic damage due to prolonged inflammation or metabolic imbalances, which affect how well the vagus nerve can communicate with the rest of the body.

The consequences of such damage can be far-reaching. Since the vagus nerve is intricately involved in many bodily functions, its impairment can lead to digestive issues, irregular heartbeats, and an inability to control blood pressure effectively. Even more troubling, given its role in the parasympathetic nervous system, damage can disrupt your ability to relax and recover, leading to heightened states of stress and anxiety.

Despite these challenges, the body possesses a remarkable capacity for healing and adaptation, and the vagus nerve is no exception. Emerging research and clinical practices have shown promising methods for aiding the recovery and regeneration of nerve function, offering hope to those affected.

One of the most groundbreaking areas of this research is nerve stimulation therapies, which use mild electrical impulses to encourage nerve activity and healing. Techniques such as Transcutaneous Vagus Nerve Stimulation (tVNS) have shown potential not only in alleviating symptoms but also in fostering the nerve's natural repair mechanisms. These therapies send electrical signals through the nerve, essentially 'reminding' it of its normal function, which can help speed the recovery process.

Moreover, lifestyle interventions are crucial in supporting nerve health and regeneration. Practices such as targeted physical therapy, nutritional adjustments to support nerve health, and stress reduction techniques can create an environment conducive to healing. Nutrients like B vitamins, omega-3 fatty acids, and magnesium are essential for their nerve-supportive roles. Incorporating these into your diet, along with adequate hydration and sleep, can provide the building blocks needed for nerve repair.

VAGUS NERVE STIMULATION: BENEFITS AND RISKS

In exploring vagus nerve stimulation (VNS), we're diving into a topic with vast potential to revolutionize how we approach health and wellness. VNS involves various techniques that directly or indirectly stimulate the vagus nerve, encouraging it to function optimally and enhance its ability to repair and regulate the body's systems. From electronic devices to manual methods, the spectrum of VNS is broad, each with its unique approach and potential benefits.

The most common form of VNS involves a small device implanted under the skin that sends electrical impulses to the vagus nerve at regular intervals. This method, often referred to as invasive VNS, has been used primarily to treat epilepsy and depression. The pulses generated prevent seizure activity and improve mood by altering neurotransmitter levels in the brain. Consider invasive VNS as a last resort if other treatments have not been effective, as it requires a surgical procedure.

On the other end of the spectrum are non-invasive VNS techniques, which are gaining popularity due to their ease of use and accessibility. These methods include transcutaneous VNS, where devices deliver electrical impulses through the skin at specific points, such as the ear, which houses a branch of the vagus nerve. This method has proven beneficial not only for epilepsy and depression but also for conditions like anxiety, heart disease, and inflammation-related disorders. Additionally, simple lifestyle practices like deep, slow breathing exercises, singing, and even gargling can act as natural vagus nerve stimulators, enhancing vagal tone and promoting overall well-being. We will explore these options at length in Part 5.

While the potential benefits of VNS are substantial, ranging from improved mental health to enhanced digestive function and reduced inflammation, it's crucial to approach these techniques with an informed perspective. Understanding the risks and potential side effects, as well as the safety considerations of each method, is essential for anyone considering VNS as part of their health regimen.

The risks associated with invasive VNS, for instance, include those related to the surgical procedure itself, such as infection or complications from anesthesia. Once implanted, side effects like hoarseness, throat pain, or voice changes may result from the device's proximity to the voice box. These side effects are generally mild and often improve over time as the body adjusts to the device.

The risks for noninvasive methods are considerably lower, but they still require attention. Skin irritation at the stimulation site and slight discomfort during the stimulation are the most common issues. However, these side effects are usually transient and resolve quickly after the stimulation session ends. To minimize adverse effects, follow the guidelines provided with the device, such as duration and intensity of use.

It's vital to consider individual health conditions when opting for VNS. For instance, individuals with cardiac issues should be cautious, particularly with invasive VNS, as the electrical impulses could potentially interfere with cardiac function. Before beginning any form of vagus nerve stimulation, it's wise to consult with a healthcare provider, ideally one familiar with VNS and its implications for various health conditions.

In summary, while vagus nerve stimulation (VNS) shows promise for treating various health conditions, it requires careful consideration. VNS highlights the complex relationship between medical innovation and the body's biology, offering hope and caution. As we explore vagus nerve treatments in the following chapters, maintaining this balanced perspective is essential to fully harness these therapies' potential while ensuring safety and efficacy.

PART III: OPTIMIZING BODILY SYSTEMS THROUGH VAGAL TONE

CHAPTER 6
IMPROVING DIGESTIVE FUNCTION

ADDRESSING DISORDERS, NUTRIENT ABSORPTION, MOTILITY AND HUNGER SIGNALING

The digestive system is a star player, fueling the entire body's activities and impacting everything from your mood to your immune system. Isn't it curious that a nerve, which doesn't digest food at all could significantly influence its operation? The vagus nerve plays a pivotal role in how your gut functions. It serves as an information superhighway, acting as a mediator between your brain and gut. This chapter explores the fascinating dynamics of the enteric nervous system, often called your body's "second brain," and reveals how the vagus nerve governs gut health, ultimately affecting overall well-being.

THE ENTERIC NERVOUS SYSTEM: THE VAGUS NERVE'S ROLE IN GUT HEALTH

Imagine a complex network of over 100 million neurons lining your gastrointestinal tract, operating independently yet harmoniously with your central nervous system. This network is your enteric nervous system (ENS), a vast and intricate neural network embedded in the gut lining, from the esophagus to the rectum. Often called the "second brain," the ENS not only controls digestion, it also communicates with the brain to affect a wide range of bodily functions. It's a clear example of how the body's systems are interconnected, with gut health profoundly influencing emotional and physical health.

The ENS operates semi-autonomously, with the vagus nerve playing a significant role as a communication bridge between your gut and brain. This relationship is vital for maintaining digestive efficiency and emotional balance. For instance, when you feel "butterflies" in your stomach before giving a speech, your ENS reacts to signals from both your brain and vagus nerve. This reaction directly results from the gut-brain connection, where emotional stress triggers a physical response in the gut. This example illustrates the vagus nerve's profound impact on gut health and overall well-being.

The vagus nerve functions like a two-way radio, constantly sending and receiving messages that affect gut function. It carries signals from the brain to the gut, influencing the release of digestive enzymes and managing muscle contractions that churn food and propel it along the digestive tract. Conversely, it sends information from the gut back to the brain, providing feedback on hunger, fullness, and the general state of the digestive system. This bi-directional communication is crucial for maintaining a balanced internal environment, allowing your body to respond adaptively to various digestive needs.

Impact on Digestion and Appetite

One of the vagus nerve's primary roles in the digestive system is to ensure that the food you consume is broken down and absorbed efficiently. It controls the production of stomach acid and digestive enzymes, essential for breaking down food into nutrients your body can absorb. If the vagus nerve's function is impaired, it can lead to digestive issues like bloating, indigestion, or even malnutrition, as your body might not be able to extract all the nutrients it needs from food.

Moreover, the vagus nerve plays a significant role in regulating appetite. It sends signals to your brain to indicate whether you're hungry or full, which helps inform your eating behaviors to prevent overeating or under-eating. Compromised signaling can harm your health. Stimulation can enhance the vagus nerve's ability to regulate these signals, leading to a healthier relationship with food and improved digestive health.

Regulation of digestive enzymes and stomach acid is essential for optimal digestion. The vagus nerve activates cells in the stomach lining to produce the right amount of stomach acid. This acid breaks down food and kills any harmful bacteria inadvertently ingested. Additionally, it signals the pancreas to release digestive enzymes, further aiding in the breakdown of fats, proteins, and carbohydrates into absorbable molecules.

Another crucial aspect of the vagus nerve's role involves managing the rhythmic contractions of the intestines, known as peristalsis. These contractions move food along the digestive tract. The vagus nerve ensures these movements are well-coordinated, consistent, and smooth, preventing issues like constipation or diarrhea.

Various types of digestive disorders, especially those involving motility issues such as chronic constipation, IBS, or gastroparesis, can often be traced back to vagal dysfunction. For individuals suffering from these conditions, therapies aimed at enhancing vagal tone can be particularly beneficial. By improving vagus nerve function, you can strengthen gut motility and alleviate some of the discomfort associated with these conditions.

Efficient nutrient absorption is crucial for overall health. Here, too, the vagus nerve plays a critical role by regulating the release of digestive enzymes, ensuring the proper breakdown of food to maximize the absorption of nutrients in the intestines. Techniques that stimulate the vagus nerve, such as deep breathing exercises or yoga, can improve its function and thus enhance your body's ability to absorb nutrients from your diet.

The vagus nerve is integral in signaling hunger and fullness to the brain, influencing appetite and eating behaviors. By regulating these signals, the vagus nerve helps maintain a healthy balance in food intake, which is crucial for weight management and metabolic health. Understanding and managing this aspect of vagal function can lead to more mindful eating patterns and healthier food relationships.

Addressing Digestive Disorders

Vagal nerve dysfunction can be a contributing factor for many people struggling with digestive disorders like IBS and GERD. Vagal stimulation techniques offer a promising avenue for alleviating these conditions. Enhancing vagal tone can improve gastrointestinal function, reduce inflammation, and ease the symptoms associated with these disorders. This approach helps manage the symptoms and addresses some of the root causes of these conditions, providing a more holistic solution to digestive health issues.

In summary, the vagus nerve's role in digestive function is broad and profound, influencing everything from enzyme secretion and gut motility to nutrient absorption and hunger signaling. By understanding and enhancing the function of this critical nerve, you can take significant strides toward improving your digestive health and overall well-being. As we explore the connections between the vagus nerve and other bodily systems in the following chapters, remember this nerve's central role in maintaining physical, emotional, and mental health simply through the enteric system.

MANAGING AND HEALING DIGESTIVE DISORDERS THROUGH VAGAL TONE IMPROVEMENT

Leaky gut syndrome might sound mysterious or questionable due to its frequent mention in alternative health circles, but it's a genuine and prevalent issue marked by increased intestinal permeability. This condition allows substances like partially digested food, toxins, and bacteria to escape into your bloodstream, leading to various health problems, including chronic inflammation, allergies, and autoimmune diseases. The vagus nerve plays a crucial role in this scenario. As a key regulator of gut integrity and immune responses, enhancing vagus nerve function can help repair the intestinal barrier and restore gut health.

Since chronic inflammation is the primary cause of leaky gut syndrome, stimulating the vagus nerve to enhance its tone supports the tightening of the intestinal junctions that become loose in leaky gut syndrome. This tightening prevents the leakage of harmful substances into the bloodstream. Techniques such as deep, slow breathing exercises, yoga, and even gentle humming can activate the vagus nerve, promoting healing in the gut lining. Over time, with consistent practice, these activities can lead to substantive improvements in gut health. Furthermore, the body's natural regenerative capabilities mean that the cells lining your gut have the potential to renew and repair themselves. Typically, the gut lining can regenerate every five to seven days. Therefore, dietary changes and lifestyle adjustments can quickly impact gut health improvement.

The vagus nerve plays a crucial role in Irritable Bowel Syndrome (IBS) and related gastrointestinal disorders. IBS, with symptoms like cramping, abdominal pain, bloating, gas, diarrhea, and constipation, indicates dysregulation in gut motility—the movement of food through the digestive tract. This dysregulation frequently traces back to vagal tone. Enhancing vagal tone through various stimulation techniques can improve gut motility, alleviating the uncomfortable and painful symptoms of IBS and similar disorders. Incorporating vagal tone exercises into a recovery plan is essential for managing these conditions effectively.

The path to healing your gut extends beyond managing symptoms—it involves comprehensive lifestyle and dietary changes that support the overall health of your digestive system. This holistic approach ensures that the improvements in vagal function and gut health are sustainable over the long term. Dietary adjustments play a vital role, including more fiber-rich foods and probiotics. The convenience of processed foods and the discomfort of adjusting dietary habits pose real challenges. It's helpful to start small and gradually incorporate more gut-friendly foods into your diet to navigate these challenges and allow your body and palate to adjust over time.

Stress management is another critical aspect of this holistic approach. Chronic stress can severely impact gut health, exacerbating symptoms of digestive disorders. Regular stress-reduction practices like meditation, mindful breathing, and gentle physical activity can significantly enhance your body's ability to manage stress, thereby supporting gut health. Integrating these practices with dietary changes can create a powerful synergy that amplifies the benefits to the vagus nerve and, by extension, your digestive system.

Monitoring your progress as you implement these changes is vital. Keeping a diary of your symptoms, diet, and stress levels can help you identify patterns and correlations between your lifestyle choices and your digestive health. Consistent monitoring helps fine-tune your approach and reinforces motivation as you see tangible improvements in your health. As you continue to apply these strategies and techniques, expect to see significant enhancements in your gut health and overall well-being, affirming the profound impact of the vagus nerve in maintaining digestive health and balance.

PROBIOTICS AND PREBIOTICS: ALLIES OF THE VAGUS NERVE

When it comes to maintaining your health, the role of the gut microbiota is impossible to ignore. This complex community of microorganisms in your digestive system profoundly impacts your overall health, influencing everything from your mood to your immune system. The vagus nerve plays a pivotal role as a mediator, shaping and being shaped by the gut microbiota. By understanding this interaction, you can harness the power of probiotics and prebiotics to support your gut health and the optimal function of your vagus nerve.

As the main component of the parasympathetic nervous system, the vagus nerve directly interacts with the gut microbiome. It sends signals that can influence the composition and activity of gut bacteria, and in return, these microbes produce metabolites that can affect the function of the vagus nerve. This two-way communication is crucial for maintaining gut balance and overall health. For example, certain beneficial bacteria produce short-chain fatty acids, which can reduce inflammation, stimulate vagal activity, enhance gut-brain communication, and promote a sense of calm and well-being.

Understanding the benefits of probiotics and prebiotics can help you appreciate their role in this complex system. Probiotics are live bacteria that add to the population of good microbes in your gut. They can help restore the balance of gut flora necessary for digestion, immune function, and even the production of some vitamins. Prebiotics, on the other hand, are non-digestible fibers that feed these beneficial bacteria, helping them to thrive and multiply. Together, probiotics and prebiotics enhance gut health, which ultimately supports the function of the vagus nerve, promoting a healthy mind-gut connection.

Not all probiotic supplements are created equal, and the effectiveness of a probiotic depends on its ability to survive the stomach's acidic environment and reach the intestines alive. Choose supplements containing well-researched strains and a delivery system that protects these bacteria until they reach your gut. Additionally, ensure that the probiotic suits your specific health needs, as different strains have different effects. For prebiotics, opt for supplements that contain a mix of fibers, such as inulin and fructooligosaccharides, to support a wide range of beneficial bacteria.

Beyond supplements, your diet is a fundamental way to support your gut microbiota and, by extension, your vagus nerve. Foods rich in probiotics include yogurt, kefir, sauerkraut, and other fermented foods. These naturally contain beneficial bacteria that can colonize your gut. Prebiotic-rich foods include garlic, onions, leeks, asparagus, and bananas, which provide the necessary fibers to feed healthy gut bacteria. Incorporating these foods into your diet can help maintain a robust and balanced gut microbiota, enhancing vagal tone and overall health.

By embracing the symbiotic relationship between probiotics, prebiotics, and the vagus nerve, you open up a natural and empowering pathway to enhanced health. By nurturing your gut microbiota, you are directly supporting the health of your vagus nerve, paving the way for improved mental, emotional, and physical health. This holistic approach to health care, focusing on the interconnectedness of body systems, offers a sustainable and effective way to enhance your quality of life and well-being.

DIETARY INFLUENCES ON VAGAL ACTIVITY: WHAT TO EAT AND AVOID

When you think about your daily meals, it's not just about satisfying hunger—it's about nurturing your body's complex systems, particularly your vagus nerve. Meal timing significantly influences vagal activation. Eating regular, balanced meals helps maintain consistent blood glucose levels, crucial for steady vagal activity. This regularity signals safety and abundance to your body, allowing the vagus nerve to support restful and digestive states rather than triggering stress responses. Adopting dietary patterns that support vagal health, such as the Mediterranean diet, enriches your system with nutrients that enhance nerve function. This diet, high in fruits, vegetables, whole grains, and healthy fats, particularly omega-3 fatty acids, supports heart health and bolsters the vagal tone, improving your overall resilience to stress and inflammation.

Understanding which foods stimulate your vagus nerve is crucial for optimal nerve function. Foods rich in probiotics, like yogurt, kefir, and sauerkraut, help maintain a healthy gut microbiome, which interacts positively with the vagus nerve to enhance its function. Omega-3 fatty acids found abundantly in fish like salmon and sardines, are critical for brain health and are linked to improved vagal tone and reduced inflammation. Magnesium, a mineral pivotal in nervous system function, can be found in leafy greens such as spinach and kale and nuts like almonds and cashews. This mineral helps relax the nervous system, thus enhancing vagal tone. Zinc, another essential nutrient in pumpkin seeds, cashews, and meat, supports brain health and mood regulation by interacting with the vagus nerve.

Conversely, some foods might dampen vagal activity. High caffeine and sugar intake, for instance, can cause spikes and crashes in blood sugar levels and energy, which can stress the body and reduce vagal tone. These substances can stimulate the sympathetic nervous system, which is responsible for the body's 'fight or flight' response, inhibiting the vagus nerve's ability to maintain calm and relaxation. Reducing these in your diet and replacing them with nutrient-rich whole foods can help maintain a more balanced and supportive environment for vagal health.

Integrating these nutritional strategies into your diet doesn't have to be overwhelming. Start by incorporating one or two vagus-nerve-friendly foods into your meals each day, and gradually adjust your meal timing to create a more regular eating schedule. Pay attention to how these changes affect your body and mood—you'll likely notice improvements in digestion, energy levels, and stress management; by making conscious choices about when and what you eat, you're taking decisive steps toward enhancing your vagal health and overall well-being.

FASTING AND THE VAGUS NERVE: A RESET FOR DIGESTIVE HEALTH

If you've been exploring ways to enhance your gut health and overall well-being, you might have stumbled upon fasting as a potential ally. Far from being just a trend or a dieting tool, fasting offers profound benefits for your digestive system and the vagus nerve, which plays a pivotal role in managing your body's relaxation responses and digestive processes. Fasting isn't merely about abstaining from food; it's a deliberate, structured pause in your eating schedule that gives your body a break, allowing it to focus on healing and rejuvenation.

Fasting influences the body and the vagus nerve by triggering what's known as the 'rest and digest' mode, a state where the body conserves energy, focuses on cellular repair and optimizes digestion. The vagus nerve mediates this state, which helps reduce heart rate and increase gastrointestinal activity. Fasting shifts your body's energy allocation away from constant digestion to other processes like autophagy (cellular cleanup) and reducing inflammation, which is crucial for long-term health. These physiological changes benefit your physical health, promote mental clarity and emotional stability, as the vagus nerve also affects mood and stress levels.

Fasting comes in various forms, each with distinct characteristics and benefits. Intermittent fasting, for example, involves cycling between periods of eating and fasting, typically allowing an eating window of eight hours followed by 16 hours of fasting. Research shows this method improves insulin sensitivity, enhances hormone function, and boosts mitochondrial health, contributing to better vagal tone. Time-restricted feeding, another popular method, limits eating to certain times of the day, syncing food intake with your circadian rhythms, thereby enhancing metabolic processes and vagal responses.

Implementing a fasting regimen with care will ensure it benefits your health without causing undue stress. Start gradually, with a shorter fasting window, and listen to your body's signals. Hydration is crucial during fasting, so increase your intake of non-caloric fluids like water and herbal teas. Also, ensure that your meals are nutrient-dense, providing all the necessary vitamins and minerals to support your body's needs. Consult a healthcare provider before starting any fasting regimen, especially if you have underlying health conditions.

By embracing fasting as a tool for health, you're not just altering your eating patterns; you're fundamentally reshaping how your body functions, promoting a better balance between energy intake and your body's natural healing processes. This chapter has explored how fasting can reset and rejuvenate your digestive health by optimizing vagal function, offering you a powerful strategy to enhance your overall well-being. As you consider integrating fasting into your lifestyle, remember it's not just about the hours you abstain from eating but about enabling your body to rest and rejuvenate, tapping into the innate healing capabilities moderated by the vagus nerve.

CHAPTER 7
STRENGTHENING MENTAL HEALTH

ADDRESSING STRESS, ANXIETY AND DEPRESSION

I n the quiet moments of self-reflection, have you ever felt as if your own body's reactions to stress and anxiety are beyond your control, as though you're watching yourself from the sidelines, unable to calm the inner turmoil? It's a universal experience, and yet, beneath the surface, a powerful ally threads through your body, largely unnoticed yet immensely influential—the vagus nerve. This chapter unveils how this nerve is pivotal not just for bodily functions but for shaping your mental landscape, offering tools to reclaim your emotional balance and break free from the cycles of stress, anxiety, and depression.

THE VAGUS NERVE'S ROLE IN MENTAL HEALTH - THE PATHWAY TO RESILIENCE

The vagus nerve plays a critical role in maintaining mental health by regulating emotional responses and contributing to the body's ability to cope with stress. By understanding the connection between the vagus nerve and mental health, we can explore various strategies to enhance vagal tone and improve overall emotional well-being.

Vagal tone, a key indicator of how well the vagus nerve is functioning, is directly linked to emotional regulation and resilience. High vagal tone is associated with an increased ability to regulate emotions, adapt to stress, and recover from psychological setbacks. It enhances your body's ability to return to calm after stress. Conversely, individuals with anxiety and depression often exhibit low vagal tone, making it challenging for them to shift out of negative emotional states.

The vagus nerve influences various neurotransmitters, including serotonin and dopamine, which play significant roles in mood regulation. Serotonin, often called the 'happiness hormone,' impacts mood, emotions, and sleep, while dopamine is linked to the brain's reward system and influences motivation, pleasure, and emotional responses. By regulating these neurotransmitters, the vagus nerve can help alleviate symptoms of depression and anxiety, providing a more stable emotional ground.

STRESS ON THE VAGUS NERVE

In acute stress situations, the body's sympathetic nervous system activates the fight-or-flight response, increasing heart rate, blood pressure, and alertness. The vagus nerve, a key component of the parasympathetic nervous system, helps counteract this response by promoting the "rest-and-digest" state, calming the body and restoring balance. This dynamic interplay ensures that the body can respond to immediate

threats while also being able to recover and return to equilibrium once the threat has passed.

While acute stress responses are short-lived and reversible,
chronic stress poses a different challenge, having a profound
and lasting impact on vagal tone and overall health. Chronic
stress occurs when the body is exposed to prolonged or
repeated stressors without sufficient recovery time, leading to
sustained activation of the stress response system.

Consequences for Mental and Physical Health

Chronic stress can significantly diminish vagal tone, weak-
ening the body's ability to engage the parasympathetic
nervous system effectively. This reduction in vagal tone
means that the vagus nerve is less capable of promoting relaxation and recovery, leaving the body in a prolonged state of
heightened arousal. As a result, individuals with low vagal
tone may find it challenging to return to a state of calm after
experiencing stress, leading to persistent feelings of anxiety
and tension.

- **Mental Health**: Low vagal tone is closely linked to
  various mental health issues, including anxiety,
  depression, and mood disorders. Without adequate
  vagal function, the regulation of critical
  neurotransmitters like serotonin and dopamine is
  impaired, exacerbating symptoms of mental health
  conditions. Individuals may experience more intense
  and prolonged episodes of anxiety and depression,
  with reduced capacity to recover from these episodes.

- **Physical Health**: Chronic stress and diminished vagal tone can also have serious physical health implications. The sustained activation of the stress response system can lead to increased inflammation, weakened immune function, and greater susceptibility to illnesses. Conditions such as cardiovascular disease, gastrointestinal disorders, and metabolic syndrome are more likely to develop in individuals with chronic stress and low vagal tone.

A detrimental feedback loop often develops between stress and vagal tone. Chronic stress decreases vagal tone, making it harder for the body to return to a state of calm. This perpetuates a cycle where the individual becomes more susceptible to stress, further reducing vagal tone and exacerbating mental and physical health issues.

Recent studies have highlighted the critical role of the vagus nerve in managing stress responses and its potential as a target for therapeutic interventions. Research has shown that individuals with higher vagal tone exhibit greater emotional stability and resilience to stress, while those with lower vagal tone are more prone to stress-related disorders.

ANXIETY AND THE VAGUS NERVE

The vagus nerve plays a crucial role in regulating the autonomic nervous system, which controls involuntary bodily functions, including heart rate, digestion, and respiratory rate. When the body perceives a threat, the sympathetic nervous system triggers the fight-or-flight response, resulting in increased heart rate, rapid breathing, and heightened alertness. In contrast, the parasympathetic nervous system, mediated by the vagus nerve, promotes a state of calm and relaxation.

In individuals with anxiety disorders, the balance between these two systems is often disrupted. Low vagal tone, which indicates reduced activity of the vagus nerve, is commonly observed in those suffering from chronic anxiety. This imbalance means that the parasympathetic nervous system is less effective in counteracting the fight-or-flight response, leading to prolonged periods of heightened arousal and anxiety.

Relationship Between Low Vagal Tone and Anxiety Disorders

Research has shown a strong correlation between low vagal tone and various anxiety disorders, including generalized anxiety disorder (GAD), panic disorder, and social anxiety disorder. Low vagal tone results in diminished regulatory capacity of the vagus nerve, making it difficult for individuals to return to a state of calm after experiencing stress or anxiety triggers. This persistent state of arousal can exacerbate anxiety symptoms and contribute to a cycle of chronic anxiety.

The vagus nerve influences several physiological processes that are directly related to anxiety symptoms:

- **Heart Rate Variability (HRV)**: Low vagal tone is associated with reduced HRV, indicating less flexibility in the autonomic nervous system's ability to adapt to stress. Lower HRV is a marker of poor parasympathetic function and is commonly found in individuals with anxiety disorders.

- **Respiratory Rate**: Anxiety often leads to rapid, shallow breathing. The vagus nerve helps regulate breathing patterns, and low vagal tone can result in inefficient respiratory control, perpetuating feelings of anxiety.
- **Digestive Function**: The vagus nerve also plays a role in regulating digestion. Low vagal tone can lead to gastrointestinal issues, such as irritable bowel syndrome (IBS), which are often comorbid with anxiety disorders.

DEPRESSION AND THE VAGUS NERVE

Depression is a complex mental health disorder characterized by persistent feelings of sadness, loss of interest or pleasure, and various physical and cognitive symptoms. Recent research has highlighted the significant role of the vagus nerve in depression, particularly through its influence on vagal tone and neurotransmitter regulation.

Relationship Between Low Vagal Tone and Depressive Symptoms

Low vagal tone is a key factor in the development and persistence of depressive symptoms. Vagal tone refers to the activity of the vagus nerve and its ability to regulate the body's physiological state. When vagal tone is low, the body's ability to manage stress and maintain emotional stability is compromised, leading to several issues that contribute to depression:

- **Reduced Resilience to Stress**: Low vagal tone weakens the parasympathetic nervous system's ability to counteract the stress response, leaving individuals more susceptible to the negative effects of chronic stress. This prolonged exposure to stress can exacerbate depressive symptoms, making it difficult for individuals to recover from stressful events.
- **Increased Inflammation**: The vagus nerve plays a critical role in regulating the body's inflammatory response. Low vagal tone is associated with higher levels of systemic inflammation, which has been linked to the development and severity of depression. Chronic inflammation can negatively affect brain function and mood, contributing to depressive symptoms.
- **Poor Heart Rate Variability (HRV)**: HRV is a measure of the variation in time between heartbeats and is an indicator of autonomic nervous system flexibility. Low HRV, often seen in individuals with low vagal tone, is associated with greater difficulty in adapting to stress and a higher risk of depression.

Neurotransmitter Imbalances Linked to Vagal Dysfunction

The vagus nerve significantly influences the regulation of neurotransmitters, which are chemicals that transmit signals in the brain and play a vital role in mood regulation. Low vagal tone can lead to imbalances in these neurotransmitters, contributing to the development and persistence of depression.

- **Serotonin**: Often referred to as the "happiness hormone," serotonin is crucial for regulating mood, sleep, and appetite. The majority of the body's serotonin is produced in the gut, with the vagus nerve serving as a communication pathway between the gut and the brain. Low vagal tone can disrupt this communication, leading to reduced serotonin levels and contributing to depressive symptoms.
- **Dopamine**: Dopamine is involved in the brain's reward system and affects motivation, pleasure, and emotional regulation. Low vagal tone can impair the regulation of dopamine, leading to a lack of motivation, anhedonia (inability to feel pleasure), and other depressive symptoms.
- **Norepinephrine**: This neurotransmitter plays a role in attention, arousal, and the stress response. Dysregulation of norepinephrine due to low vagal tone can result in increased stress sensitivity and depressive symptoms.

Understanding the connection between low vagal tone and neurotransmitter imbalances highlights the importance of maintaining healthy vagal function for mental health. Enhancing vagal tone can help regulate neurotransmitter levels, reduce inflammation, and improve resilience to stress, all of which are critical for managing and alleviating depressive symptoms.

In summary, low vagal tone significantly contributes to the development and persistence of depressive symptoms through its effects on stress resilience, inflammation, and neurotransmitter regulation. By recognizing the role of the vagus nerve in depression, we can better understand the underlying mechanisms of this complex disorder and explore effective strategies to enhance vagal tone and improve mental health. The following sections will delve deeper into specific techniques and lifestyle practices to support vagal health and manage depression effectively.

BIOHACKING AND HOLISTIC PRACTICES FOR MENTAL HEALTH

The vagus nerve plays a significant role in mental health by regulating neurotransmitters like serotonin and dopamine, which impact mood and emotional stability. Optimal vagus nerve function supports a balanced emotional state, enhancing resilience against stress and reducing the likelihood of anxiety and depression. Dysfunction, however, can lead to mood swings and emotional distress.

A holistic approach to treating mood disorders involves more than symptom management. It integrates practices that enhance vagal tone and improve overall mental health. While antidepressants adjust neurotransmitter levels, incorporating vagal stimulation techniques—such as controlled breathing, yoga, and gentle electric stimulation—can enhance these effects by improving vagal tone. This combination of traditional medical treatments and vagus nerve activation techniques, detailed later in the book, can alleviate symptoms more effectively and contribute to long-term wellness.

Biohacking Your Nervous System for Calm

Biohacking, a powerful method of understanding and enhancing your body's functions, is a holistic approach to treating ailments like stress, anxiety, and depression. It involves making small, gradual adjustments to achieve significant health improvements by considering the entire ecosystem of your body.

Key strategies include:

- **Nutrition**: Consuming omega-3 fatty acids and probiotics supports neural health, promoting better brain function and emotional stability.
- **Exercise**: Engaging in activities that stimulate neurogenesis, such as aerobic exercises and yoga, enhances cognitive function and reduces stress.
- **Technology**: Devices that monitor heart rate variability (HRV) or track sleep patterns provide real-time data, helping you understand how different activities affect your nervous system and stress levels. This information allows you to make informed adjustments to your lifestyle for better stress management.

Simple lifestyle adjustments can also yield profound benefits. Mindfulness meditation, exposure to nature, and grounding activities like walking barefoot on grass can significantly enhance vagal tone and reduce stress responses. Combining these techniques may initially feel overwhelming, but biohacking's adaptability and personalization allow for a tailored approach that evolves with your needs.

Biohacking isn't just about reducing moments of anxiety or stress; it's about fundamentally enhancing your body's baseline state, making it more resilient and capable of handling challenges. Each small change is a step towards a calmer, more controlled nervous system, equipping you to manage stress and thrive.

This holistic approach to mental health, emphasizing the integration of body and mind therapies, highlights the vagus nerve's potential as a critical treatment target. By fostering better gut health, enhancing vagal tone, and incorporating supportive lifestyle changes, you can address mood disorder symptoms and build a foundation for lasting emotional and physical health. Each step forward moves you towards a more balanced and fulfilling life, guided by the vagus nerve on your journey to wellness.

CHAPTER 8

ELEVATING QUALITY OF LIFE
ADDRESSING CHRONIC PAIN AND INFLAMMATION

W hen you wake up with stiffness and pain, it's not just your body that feels burdened—your spirit does, too. Chronic inflammation and pain are more than just annoyances; they're signals from your body indicating that something deeper needs healing. The vagus nerve is central to easing these persistent issues. In this chapter, we'll delve into how the vagus nerve can help manage chronic pain and inflammation, providing practical tips to harness its power for your overall well-being.

THE VAGUS NERVE AND CHRONIC INFLAMMATION: GETTING TO THE ROOT OF CHRONIC PAIN

At the core of your body's response to inflammation lies the vagus nerve, which wields the power to sense and quell inflammation through a remarkable mechanism known as the cholinergic anti-inflammatory pathway. Picture this pathway as a high-speed road, where the vagus nerve sends rapid signals that directly inhibit the production of cytokines, the proteins responsible for inflammation. The vagus nerve releases acetylcholine, a neurotransmitter that actively targets immune cells producing these inflammatory proteins. Doing so effectively prevents the systemic spread of inflammation, reduces local swelling and pain, and mitigates the risk of conditions linked to chronic inflammation, such as heart disease and arthritis.

For many, chronic pain is relentless, ebbing and flowing but never fully receding. This type of pain is frequently rooted in persistent inflammation—a fire that the body mistakenly keeps feeding. The vagus nerve's role in modulating this inflammatory response offers hope. Enhancing vagal tone through stimulation techniques can dampen the inflammatory signals and, thus, the associated pain.

Imagine a future where inflammation management is as straightforward as wearing a device that modulates nerve activity gently. This idea may sound like science fiction, but it is happening today due to the advancement of bioelectronic medicine. Vagus nerve stimulation (VNS) devices, both non-invasive and implantable, are at the forefront of this innovation, offering new hope to those suffering from inflammatory conditions. These devices deliver electrical impulses to the vagus nerve, enhancing its ability to regulate the immune response and prevent excessive inflammation.

While technology offers novel solutions, managing chronic inflammation lies in lifestyle choices. Simple, daily actions can profoundly influence the inflammatory process. Engaging in regular physical activity, ensuring adequate and restful sleep, and incorporating stress reduction techniques like meditation or yoga can all enhance vagal tone and reduce inflammation. Moreover, dietary choices play a pivotal role. Integrating anti-inflammatory foods such as leafy greens, fatty fish rich in omega-3 fatty acids, and turmeric while reducing inflammatory agents like sugar and processed foods can significantly bolster your body's defenses against inflammation.

Clinical Evidence: Vagus Nerve Stimulation (VNS) in Action

Clinical research increasingly supports the promise of vagus nerve stimulation (VNS) in managing chronic inflammation, moving beyond anecdotal evidence. Studies have shown that targeted VNS can significantly reduce symptoms in conditions like rheumatoid arthritis and Crohn's disease, offering relief where traditional medications fell short.

A landmark study published in the *Proceedings of the National Academy of Sciences* demonstrated that patients with rheumatoid arthritis who had not responded to standard treatments experienced a marked reduction in their symptoms following regular sessions of vagus nerve stimulation. Koopman et al. (2016) conducted a double-blind, randomized control trial with 17 patients, highlighting a significant decrease in inflammatory markers such as TNF-alpha and IL-6 after consistent VNS treatment. These reductions accompanied improved joint function and a substantial decrease in pain scores.

Furthermore, a review by Bonaz, Sinniger, and Pellissier (2017) in *Frontiers in Neuroscience* highlighted the efficacy of

VNS in reducing inflammation in patients with Crohn's disease. The review noted that VNS helped decrease the levels of pro-inflammatory cytokines and improved the clinical symptoms of Crohn's disease patients, suggesting its potential as a therapeutic approach for inflammatory bowel diseases (Bonaz, Sinniger, & Pellissier, 2017).

These findings not only illuminate the potential of VNS as a treatment modality but also underscore the vagus nerve's central role in controlling inflammation and, by extension, pain. Understanding and leveraging the power of the vagus nerve can be transformative in navigating the complexities of chronic pain and inflammation. Its ability to modulate the body's inflammatory response offers a pathway to relief. It aligns with a broader vision of health that embraces the body's inherent capacities for self-regulation and healing.

THE VAGUS NERVE AND PAIN PERCEPTION: PATHWAYS TO RELIEF

One of the vagus nerve's more surprising attributes is its ability to subtly shape how you perceive and respond to pain. Its ability to influence pain perception is deeply intertwined with its role in the central nervous system, modulating pain signals before they reach the brain. This modulation is crucial because it can significantly alter your experience of pain, potentially reducing the intensity of the pain signals and offering a more manageable sensation.

The vagus nerve's impact on pain perception is rooted in its ability to release neurotransmitters that calm inflammation and decrease pain signals. For example, by increasing levels of neurotransmitters like GABA, the nerve can dampen the excitability of neurons that would typically escalate pain signals. This mechanism provides a buffer against the raw edge of chronic pain, which can be a relentless force in your daily life. Furthermore, the vagus nerve can enhance the release of endorphins, the body's natural painkillers, which help elevate your mood and reduce pain perception, making it a natural and holistic approach to pain management.

Neuroplasticity, the brain's ability to reorganize itself by forming new neural connections, is pivotal in managing chronic pain. Chronic pain can lead to maladaptive changes in the brain's neural pathways, essentially 'rewiring' the brain to be more sensitive to pain signals. This heightened sensitivity can make even mild stimuli feel excruciating. However, the vagus nerve, through its extensive network in the brain, has the potential to influence these neural pathways. Promoting positive neuroplastic changes can help diminish the brain's sensitivity to pain signals, relieving the constant discomfort that characterizes chronic pain conditions.

Non-Pharmacological Pain Management

Vagal nerve stimulation (VNS) presents a compelling, non-pharmacological approach to pain management. This method uses devices that deliver electrical impulses to the vagus nerve, enhancing its tone and function. The beauty of VNS lies in its ability to provide pain relief without the side effects of pain medications, such as dependency or gastrointestinal issues. For individuals grappling with chronic pain, VNS offers a promising alternative that not only alleviates pain but also enhances overall well-being by improving sleep, mood, and energy levels.

Integrating vagal stimulation with other holistic practices can amplify its efficacy in managing pain. For instance, combining VNS with yoga and mindfulness meditation can create a synergistic effect that enhances vagal tone and reduces pain perception. These integrative approaches address pain not just at a physiological level but also at an emotional and psychological level, providing a comprehensive strategy for managing conditions like fibromyalgia and migraine headaches.

Adopting an anti-inflammatory diet supports the vagus nerve and aids in pain management. Foods high in omega-3 fatty acids, antioxidants, and phytonutrients reduce inflammation in the body, including the nervous system. This diet helps control inflammation that contributes to chronic pain and strengthens the vagus nerve's ability to manage pain.

As this chapter closes, remember that managing chronic pain is not just about dulling the discomfort. It is about nurturing the intricate systems that influence pain perception and response. The vagus nerve, with its profound connection to the mind and body, offers a pathway to relief despite the challenges posed by chronic pain conditions. Next, we'll explore the vagus nerve's role in enhancing immune function, further expanding on this remarkable nerve's influence on health and well-being.

CHAPTER 9
BOOSTING IMMUNITY
GUARDING YOUR HEALTH AND SLEEP

I magine your immune system is a well-trained security detail, patrolling and protecting your body from potential threats like infections and diseases. The vagus nerve acts as the commander of this detail, using its extensive network to communicate and direct immune responses efficiently. Through its powerful influence on the immune system, the vagus nerve is a critical ally in your body's defense mechanism, enhancing your ability to resist and recover from illnesses.

THE VAGUS NERVE AND DISEASE RESISTANCE

Previously, you learned about the cholinergic anti-inflammatory pathway, where the vagus nerve helps regulate inflammation. Let's delve deeper into how this works from the perspective of the immune response. When the body detects an infection or inflammation, this pathway activates as a reflex to reduce the production of cytokines, proteins that can cause inflammation if left unchecked. Immune cell receptors bind to acetylcholine, the neurotransmitter released by the vagus nerve, instructing the body to "turn down" the inflammatory response. This mechanism not only prevents excessive inflammation, which can lead to autoimmune diseases but also maintains the balance and health of your immune system, ensuring it functions optimally to protect you from various illnesses.

Enhancing the tone of your vagus nerve—its readiness and ability to send effective signals—plays a pivotal role in your body's defense against diseases. A well-toned vagus nerve can quickly mobilize your immune system's response to infections, reducing the duration and severity of illnesses. The mechanisms here involve intricate biochemical signals where the vagus nerve influences the release of various hormones and neurotransmitters that regulate immune cells. For instance, the hormone oxytocin, which the vagus nerve helps release, has been shown to have anti-inflammatory effects and to modulate immune responses. Maintaining a high vagal tone enhances your body's ability to fend off pathogens and recover more swiftly from illnesses.

Vagus Nerve and Autoimmune Diseases

Navigating the complex waters of autoimmune diseases, where the body mistakenly attacks its healthy cells, often feels like an uphill battle. These conditions are multifactorial, involving genetic, environmental, and immunological factors. While the breakdown of the cholinergic anti-inflammatory pathway is not the sole cause of autoimmune diseases, it can significantly contribute to immune response dysregulation.

Impairment or dysfunction of this pathway can lead to an inability to properly regulate inflammation, potentially resulting in chronic inflammatory states and autoimmune conditions. Strict control of inflammation in autoimmune conditions is necessary to prevent damage to healthy tissues.

Emerging research suggests that enhancing the cholinergic anti-inflammatory pathway could be a promising approach to managing autoimmune diseases. By leveraging this pathway, it may be possible to better control inflammation, thereby preventing damage to healthy tissues. Within this challenging landscape, the vagus nerve emerges as a critical communicator and potential peacemaker. With its extensive reach and influence over various bodily functions, the vagus nerve plays a pivotal role in modulating immune responses, offering new insights and hope in managing autoimmune conditions.

Holistic Approaches to Boost Immunity

Given its significant role in modulating immune responses, activating your vagus nerve through stimulation techniques has emerged as a promising therapeutic strategy for treating autoimmune diseases. It is also a promising complementary treatment option for those with compromised immune systems, such as those undergoing radiation or chemo-therapy..

Supporting your vagus nerve and, by extension, your immune system doesn't always require high-tech stimulation devices. Simple, holistic approaches can also effectively bolster your immune defense. Dietary choices play a crucial role; incorporating foods rich in omega-3 fatty acids, antioxidants, and vitamins can enhance vagal tone and immune function. Engaging regularly in activities that activate the parasympathetic nervous system, detailed at length in Part 4 of this book, provides ample opportunity to gently enhance vagal tone, thereby boosting your body's resilience against pathogens and improving overall immune function.

While holistic methods offer numerous ways to reduce stress and support your immune system, you cannot overstate the importance of quality sleep. Sleep is crucial in maintaining a strong immune response, allowing the body to repair and rejuvenate. The next chapter will delve into the critical connection between the vagus nerve and sleep quality, offering insights into cultivating better sleep habits for overall health and well-being.

THE VAGUS NERVE AND SLEEP QUALITY: CULTIVATING SOOTHING SLUMBER

In the delicate ballet of nightly rejuvenation, where your body and mind surrender to the restorative powers of sleep, the vagus nerve emerges as a subtle yet powerful conductor. Its role in regulating sleep patterns extends beyond mere timing; it influences the quality and depth of your slumber, orchestrating a symphony of physiological processes that restore balance and wellness in every cell of your body. Understanding the physiological mechanisms by which vagal tone impacts sleep quality can transform your approach to sleep, turning restless nights into peaceful slumber.

The vagus nerve primarily interacts with your body's sleep regulation mechanisms by influencing neurotransmitters and hormones associated with sleep cycles. For instance, it helps regulate levels of serotonin and melatonin, two critical components of healthy sleep. Serotonin, often associated with mood regulation, also plays a crucial role in setting the stage for sleep. As evening approaches, the body converts serotonin to melatonin, the hormone that cues your body that it's time to wind down. A well-toned vagus nerve ensures this conversion process runs smoothly, promoting timely and adequate melatonin production for restful sleep.

Moreover, the vagus nerve's ability to promote relaxation through the parasympathetic nervous system (your rest and digest system) directly contributes to your ability to fall and stay asleep. Activating this system through vagal stimulation techniques like deep breathing or gentle yoga before bedtime can help quiet the mind and prepare the body for sleep, leading to deeper and more restorative sleep cycles.

Sleep Quality and Inflammation, Pain and Immunity

Quality of sleep closely correlates with inflammation levels in your body. During deep, restorative sleep, your body enters a state of significant healing and regeneration, where it can effectively regulate inflammatory responses. Poor sleep quality disrupts this process, often leading to elevated levels of pro-inflammatory cytokines. These inflammatory markers not only exacerbate existing conditions like arthritis or asthma but can also set the stage for a host of chronic diseases, including cardiovascular diseases and diabetes. By improving sleep quality through vagal activation, you not only enhance your nightly rest but also contribute to lowering systemic inflammation, thereby protecting against these chronic conditions.

The relationship between sleep quality and pain is another critical area influenced by the vagus nerve. Poor sleep can significantly lower your pain threshold, making you more sensitive to pain stimuli, which creates a vicious cycle, especially for those suffering from chronic pain conditions. Pain disrupts sleep, and inadequate sleep exacerbates pain. You can break this cycle by improving vagal tone and, thus, sleep quality. Techniques that enhance vagal activity, such as mindfulness meditation or progressive muscle relaxation at bedtime, have proven effective in improving sleep and reducing pain sensitivity, offering a dual benefit for chronic pain patients.

The immune system also relies heavily on quality sleep for optimal function. During sleep, your body releases cytokines crucial for fighting infections and inflammation. The vagus nerve plays a role here, too, regulating the production of these cytokines to ensure that your immune system functions efficiently without becoming overactive, which could lead to autoimmunity. Enhancing sleep quality through vagal stimulation ensures your body maintains this delicate balance, optimizing your immune response and keeping you healthier overall.

Practical Techniques to Enhance Sleep

Direct vagal stimulation can be a game-changer for those struggling with insomnia or other sleep disorders. Techniques like transcutaneous vagus nerve stimulation (tVNS) before bedtime can increase parasympathetic activity and promote relaxation, making falling and staying asleep easier. Many have found these methods to be effective alternatives to sleep medications, which can have undesirable side effects and contribute to dependency.

In addition to these practical techniques, it's essential to consider the environmental and behavioral factors contributing to sleep quality. Establishing a regular sleep routine, making your sleeping environment comfortable and free from disturbances, and limiting exposure to blue light from screens before bed are all critical components of good sleep hygiene. Combining these practices with vagal stimulation techniques creates a comprehensive approach to improving sleep that can significantly enhance your overall health and well-being.

In this exploration of the vagus nerve's role in sleep, we've uncovered how its regulation of neurotransmitters, anti-inflammatory actions, and influence on pain and immune function all converge to impact the quality of your sleep. By understanding and leveraging these mechanisms, you can transform your approach to sleep from frustration or resignation to empowerment and renewal. As we close this chapter, remember that each night offers a new opportunity to nurture your body and mind through the simple yet profound act of sleeping, guided by your vagus nerve's quiet but powerful influence.

CHAPTER 10
ENHANCING HOLISTIC RECOVERY

ACCELERATING HEALING, BALANCING HORMONES, OVERCOMING ADDICTION, AND TRAUMA

I n the journey toward holistic recovery, the vagus nerve emerges as a pivotal player, orchestrating responses that promote healing from various physical and emotional challenges. Whether recovering from illness, balancing hormones, overcoming addiction, or navigating post-traumatic growth, the vagus nerve acts as a silent healer, enhancing your body's resilience and capacity for renewal. This chapter explores how improving vagal tone can bolster your immune system, regulate hormones, support addiction recovery, and facilitate emotional healing, setting the stage for future chapters that will offer comprehensive strategies to reclaim your health and well-being.

IMPROVING RECOVERY SPEED FROM ILLNESSES

Imagine your immune system as a well-trained army guarding your body against the onslaught of infections and diseases. Now, imagine the vagus nerve as the experienced general of this army, equipped with strategies that enhance the efficiency and responsiveness of your immune defenses. Improved vagal tone means this general is highly effective, able to quickly mobilize your immune cells to the sites of infection or injury, thereby accelerating your recovery.

Scientific studies underscore the significance of high vagal tone in reducing the body's time to heal. By carefully regulating inflammation, the body's natural response to injury or infection, the vagus nerve can prevent it from becoming excessive, thus fostering quicker healing. The vagus nerve also plays a crucial role in immune modulation through several other mechanisms. Beyond the cholinergic anti-inflammatory pathway, it influences immune function via neuroimmune modulation, HPA axis regulation, the microbiome-gut-brain axis, and direct cellular communication. By interacting with the hypothalamic-pituitary-adrenal (HPA) axis, the vagus nerve helps regulate cortisol levels, which affects immune responses. High cortisol levels, often resulting from chronic stress, can suppress the immune system, making the body more susceptible to infections and slowing the healing process. By regulating cortisol, the vagus nerve helps to maintain a balanced immune response. It also plays a crucial role in maintaining gut health, influencing the immune system through the microbiome-gut-brain axis. Additionally, the vagus nerve can directly communicate with immune cells, such as macrophages, dendritic cells, and T cells, enhancing their activity and function. These combined actions help the body maintain homeostasis, efficiently respond to infections and injuries, and prevent excessive inflammation, thus speeding up recovery and promoting overall health.

Numerous clinical studies support the practical applications of vagus nerve stimulation (VNS) in accelerating recovery speed. Research has explored the potential of VNS as an adjunct therapy for COVID-19, demonstrating its ability to attenuate inflammation by modulating cholinergic anti-inflammatory pathways. This modulation helps to reduce the cytokine storm associated with severe COVID-19 cases, thereby promoting quicker recovery and better outcomes for patients with severe respiratory infections.

In the context of surgical recovery, clinical trials have shown that VNS can significantly decrease inflammation and expedite the healing of surgical wounds. By regulating the body's immune response and reducing excessive inflammation, VNS supports more efficient tissue repair, leading to faster post-operative recovery. Studies have highlighted that VNS not only helps in managing pain and inflammation but also enhances overall healing processes, resulting in improved recovery speeds.

HORMONAL BALANCE AND REGULATION

In the intricate dance of your body's systems, the vagus nerve plays a pivotal role not only in your immediate responses to stress but also in the delicate balance of your hormones. This nerve, wandering and wise, connects to your endocrine system, influencing the secretion and regulation of critical hormones like cortisol, known for its role in stress response, and oxytocin, often celebrated as the hormone of relaxation and connection. Understanding this connection opens up new pathways to managing your hormonal health, crucial for everything from your mood to your metabolism.

When you feel stressed, your adrenal glands release cortisol. This hormone is essential for managing stress, but constant elevation in its levels can lead to a host of health issues, including anxiety, weight gain, and even heart disease. Here, the vagus nerve steps in as a regulator, capable of modulating the release of cortisol by stimulating the parasympathetic nervous system—the calm counter to the stress-induced fight-or-flight response. Enhancing vagal tone can help your body temper its cortisol response, maintaining a more balanced state that supports overall well-being.

Oxytocin, on the other hand, enhances feelings of trust, empathy, and bonding and can also reduce stress. The vagus nerve stimulates the release of this hormone, reinforcing its role in calming the body and promoting positive social inter-actions. It's a beautiful feedback loop; as you engage in behav-iors that stimulate the vagus nerve, such as deep breathing or social bonding, you enhance your vagal tone and encourage your body to release more oxytocin, deepening your sense of calm and connection.

Insulin, a hormone produced by the pancreas, is crucial for regulating blood sugar levels. The vagus nerve helps modulate insulin secretion, influencing your body's ability to maintain stable energy levels and preventing conditions like diabetes.

Similarly, the thyroid gland, a small butterfly-shaped organ in your neck, plays a significant role in your metabolism, energy levels, and hormonal health. The vagus nerve influences thyroid function by regulating the release of thyroid hormones, which help control your metabolic rate. An imbalance in these hormones can lead to conditions like hypothyroidism or hyperthyroidism, affecting your energy levels and overall health. Maintaining a healthy vagal tone can support balanced thyroid function and ensure your thyroid responds appropriately to your body's needs, promoting overall metabolic health and effective weight management.

THE VAGUS NERVE'S ROLE IN ADDICTION RECOVERY

In the realm of addiction recovery, where every step forward is both a challenge and a victory, the vagus nerve emerges as a potent ally, offering new hope and methods to those seeking freedom from the grips of dependency. This nerve's influence extends deep into the brain's reward systems, primarily involving neurotransmitters like dopamine, which plays a crucial role in the cycle of addiction. By understanding and harnessing the power of the vagus nerve, you can tap into its ability to restore balance to these systems, potentially transforming the landscape of addiction treatment.

Dopamine, often known as the 'feel-good' neurotransmitter, is central to the experience of pleasure and reward. In the context of addiction, dopamine pathways can become skewed, with substance use or addictive behaviors leading to excessive dopamine releases, reinforcing the cycle of addiction. Here, the vagus nerve can play a corrective role. Its extensive network of fibers can modulate neurotransmitter release and reactivity in the brain, promoting a more balanced dopamine output. This modulation helps to stabilize mood and reduce the dopamine-driven reward-seeking behavior commonly seen in addiction. Enhanced vagal tone, achieved through various stimulation techniques, can thus help recalibrate the reward system, making it less responsive to addictive substances and more responsive to natural rewards.

Research has shown that vagus nerve stimulation (VNS) can significantly impact addiction recovery by altering brain activity and reducing cravings. For instance, a study by the University of Texas at Dallas demonstrated that VNS could reduce drug-seeking behaviors in cocaine-addicted rats by altering synaptic plasticity between the prefrontal cortex and the amygdala. This process, known as "extinction learning," helps rewire the brain to reduce the association between drug-related cues and rewards, thereby decreasing cravings and relapse rates.

Additionally, VNS has been used to alleviate the severe withdrawal symptoms associated with opioid addiction. The NSS-2 Bridge device, approved by the FDA, is designed to manage opioid withdrawal by reducing symptoms such as nausea and anxiety. Clinical studies have shown that patients using this device experienced significant reductions in withdrawal symptoms, making it easier for them to transition to long-term recovery programs. In a clinical trial, 88% of patients successfully transitioned to medication-assisted therapy after using the device for five days, highlighting its effectiveness in supporting addiction recovery.

These findings underscore the transformative potential of vagus nerve stimulation in the treatment of addiction. By modulating brain activity and reducing withdrawal symptoms, VNS offers a promising adjunct therapy that can enhance the efficacy of traditional addiction treatments and support long-term recovery.

THE VAGUS NERVE'S ROLE IN POST-TRAUMATIC GROWTH

When life throws its worst at us, the aftermath can sometimes lead to profound personal growth. This process, known as post-traumatic growth, refers to the positive psychological changes that occur after struggling with highly challenging life circumstances. It's not just about returning to your baseline but evolving to a place where you find new meaning, strength, and resilience. Understanding this can be a beacon of hope, showing that a path to transformation exists through the shadow of trauma.

The vagus nerve, your body's natural calm mediator, is crucial in navigating the post-traumatic path. It plays a pivotal role in emotional regulation by controlling the parasympathetic nervous system, acting as the brake to your body's stress response. When you experience trauma, your body's fight-or-flight response can go into overdrive, making you feel constantly on edge. Here, the vagus nerve steps in, helping to slow your heart rate, decrease blood pressure, and promote a calming effect.

Enhancing the tone of this nerve can significantly influence your ability to manage post-traumatic stress and foster emotional resilience, which is essential for achieving post-traumatic growth. By strengthening your vagal tone through practices like deep breathing, meditation, and mindful movement, you can support your body in finding calm amidst the chaos. This journey of recovery and growth is deeply personal, and nurturing your vagus nerve can be a powerful ally in reclaiming your peace and building a stronger, more resilient self.

The relationship between enhanced vagal tone and increased post-traumatic growth is not just anecdotal; research supports it. Studies have demonstrated that individuals with higher vagal tone exhibit greater emotional flexibility and lower levels of stress hormones, which are crucial in adapting to life post-trauma. For example, one study observed that participants who engaged in regular practices that stimulate the vagus nerve, such as meditation and yoga, reported higher levels of post-traumatic growth, including a greater appreciation of life and deeper personal relationships. These findings underscore the transformative potential of nurturing the vagus nerve in the aftermath of trauma. By incorporating practices that enhance vagal tone, you're not just surviving; you're paving the way for thriving, turning your past pains into stepping stones for growth.

This chapter aims to educate and inspire you to view your recovery journey through a lens of growth and possibility. As we continue to explore the multifaceted roles of the vagus nerve in subsequent chapters, keep in mind the profound impact that fostering this nerve can have on overcoming trauma and embarking on a fulfilling path of post-traumatic growth.

As we conclude Chapter 10 and Part 3 of our journey, we've explored the profound impact the vagus nerve has on optimizing various bodily systems, from enhancing immune function and hormonal balance to supporting addiction recovery and fostering post-traumatic growth. Understanding the pivotal role of the vagus nerve in these areas underscores its importance in achieving holistic well-being.

But this is just the beginning. Imagine having the tools to actively influence your body's resilience and emotional healing. In the upcoming chapters of Part 4, we will dive into the therapeutic techniques and practical applications for activating and stimulating the vagus nerve. You will discover actionable strategies to harness its full potential for health and healing, transforming the theoretical knowledge into practical steps you can take every day.

Get ready to embark on a hands-on journey where you will learn how to integrate simple yet powerful practices into your routine—practices that can significantly enhance your well-being. From breathing exercises and mindful movements to innovative technologies and lifestyle adjustments, these techniques will empower you to reclaim your health and vitality.

As you turn the page to Part 4, reflect on the incredible capacity of your body to heal and grow. Embrace the upcoming chapters with curiosity and an open heart, knowing that each step forward brings you closer to a balanced, thriving life. The journey towards holistic recovery is not just about overcoming challenges—it's about evolving into a stronger, more resilient version of yourself. Let's take this next step together, unlocking the full potential of your vagus nerve and paving the way for lasting health and happiness.

PART IV: THERAPEUTIC TECHNIQUES FOR STIMULATING THE VAGUS NERVE

CHAPTER 11
BREATHING EXERCISES

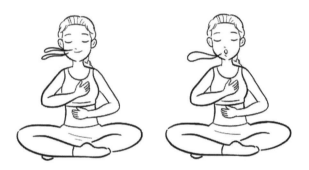

B reathing exercises are not just about inhaling and exhaling. You can use the breath as a powerful tool to activate and stimulate the vagus nerve, leading to profound physical and mental benefits. This chapter delves into various breathing techniques to enhance vagal tone, promote relaxation, and improve overall well-being. As you explore these practices, you'll learn how to integrate simple yet effective breathwork into your daily routine to support your journey toward optimal health.

BREATHING TECHNIQUES FOR VAGAL ACTIVATION: A PRACTICAL CIRCUIT

Imagine your breath as a gentle wave lapping against the shores of your nervous system, and each inhale draws in calmness, each exhale pushing out tension. Far from just poetic imagery, this is the essence of how deep, slow breathing can activate your vagus nerve, the tranquil pathway to relaxation and stress reduction. When you engage in deep breathing, you signal to your brain to activate the vagus nerve, which down-regulates the stress response and up-regulates the relaxation response. This physiological change is not only about feeling calm but also about encouraging a state of physical and mental recovery and resilience.

The benefits of such breath-focused exercises are vast, linking directly to improved vagal tone, which measures how effectively your body can relax and recover from stress. When your vagal tone is high, your body can relax faster after stress, which is crucial for overall health and well-being. High vagal tone improves your heart rate variability (HRV), lowers your risk of heart disease, and enhances your mood by regulating neurotransmitters like serotonin and dopamine.

Incorporating breathing exercises into your daily routine might seem daunting. Still, it can be as simple as taking a few moments to breathe deeply before a stressful meeting or to wind down before sleep. These practices are not only about improving your physical health. They also manage anxiety, enhance sleep quality, and prepare your mind and body to face challenges with a steadier hand. Whether it's a few slow breaths before you step into a challenging situation or a dedicated breathing session to close off your day, the flexibility of breathwork allows it to weave seamlessly into the fabric of your daily life.

Let's explore some specific breathing techniques you can start to reap the benefits of this calming practice immediately.

Diaphragmatic Breathing: Engaging the Core of Calm

Also known as abdominal breathing, diaphragmatic breathing is a fundamental technique that promotes full oxygen exchange while activating the vagus nerve. To practice this:

1. Find a comfortable position: Sit comfortably or lie flat on your back. Place one hand on your belly beneath your ribs and the other on your chest.
2. Inhale deeply through your nose: Allow your belly to push your hand out. Your chest should not move.
3. Exhale through pursed lips as if you were whistling: Feel the hand on your belly go in, and use it to help push all the air out.
4. Repeat this breathing pattern 3 to 10 times. Take your time with each breath.
5. Notice how you feel at the end of the session.

Box Breathing Practice: Clarity in Four Corners

Box breathing, or square breathing, is a powerful technique to help manage stress and improve concentration. Here's how to do it:

1. Inhale slowly and deeply through your nose for 4 seconds. Feel the air moving into your lungs and your abdomen expanding.
2. Hold your breath for 4 seconds. Try to avoid clenching your muscles.
3. Exhale slowly through your mouth for 4 seconds, expelling as much air as possible.
4. Hold your breath again for 4 seconds before inhaling again.
5. Repeat this process for several minutes.

4-7-8 Breathing: The Relaxing Breath

The 4-7-8 breathing technique is simple, quick, and effective at helping you relax and relieve anxiety. Here's how you can practice it:

1. Empty your lungs of air.
2. Breathe in quietly through the nose for 4 seconds.
3. Hold your breath for a count of 7 seconds.
4. Exhale forcefully through the mouth, pursing the lips, and making a "whoosh" sound for 8 seconds.
5. Repeat the cycle up to 4 times.

Resonant Breathing: Harmonizing Body and Mind

Resonant, or coherent, breathing helps to optimize your heart rate variability and induce calmness. To practice resonant breathing:

1. Inhale for 5 seconds
2. Exhale for 5 seconds.
3. This slow, rhythmic breathing helps to synchronize your heart rate and breathing pattern. Aim to complete about 5-6 breaths per minute.

Pursed Lip Breathing: Simple Relief

Pursed lip breathing is particularly effective for those with respiratory issues but also reduces stress and anxiety. Here's how to do it:

1. Breathe through your nose for 2 seconds (a little quicker than other techniques).
2. Pucker your lips as if you're going to whistle.
3. Exhale slowly through pursed lips for about 4 seconds.
4. Repeat this process as needed to relieve symptoms or stress.

By integrating these breathing techniques into your daily routine, you can take significant steps toward enhancing your vagal tone and overall well-being.

PRANAYAMA: YOGIC BREATHING FOR VAGAL BALANCE

Pranayama, the ancient art of breath control, originates from the Sanskrit words 'prana,' meaning life force, and 'ayama,' meaning extension. This practice is an integral part of yoga that focuses on enhancing and regulating the life force through specific breathing techniques. Historically, the yogis of ancient India developed pranayama, understanding the profound impact of breath control on the mind and body. They discovered that manipulating the breath could alter mental states, enhance physical health, and achieve higher states of consciousness. These breathing techniques influence the autonomic nervous system, including the vagus nerve, promoting balance and calm.

Pranayama practices are varied, each with unique benefits and methods, but all enhance vagal tone, similar to other breathing exercises. However, pranayama extends beyond simple deep breathing by incorporating timing, duration, and posture, intensifying its effects on the nervous system.

Let's explore some specific types of pranayama that you can incorporate into your daily routine to help balance your nervous system and enhance your mental clarity. When practiced regularly, these techniques can significantly boost your vagal tone, contributing to improved overall health.

Alternate Nostril Breathing (Nadi Shodhana)

This technique is known for its ability to balance the right and left hemispheres of the brain, harmonize the nervous system, and improve focus. Here's how to practice Nadi Shodhana:

1. Sit comfortably with your spine erect and shoulders relaxed.
2. Place your left hand on your knee, palm open to the sky.

3. Using your right hand, fold your index and middle fingers towards your palm, leaving your thumb, ring finger, and pinky extended.
4. Close your right nostril with your thumb and inhale slowly through the left nostril.
5. Close your left nostril with your ring finger, open your right nostril, and exhale slowly.
6. Inhale through the right nostril, close it with your thumb, open your left nostril, and exhale.
7. Continue this pattern for several minutes, focusing on your breath and the rhythm of alternating nostrils.

Bhramari (Bee Breath)

Bhramari is renowned for its immediate calming effects on the mind. It is particularly effective in releasing agitation, frustration, or anxiety.

1. Sit comfortably, closing your eyes and relaxing your face.
2. Place your index fingers on your ears, gently closing them.
3. Inhale deeply, and as you exhale, make a loud humming sound like a bee, feeling the vibration throughout your body.
4. Repeat 5-7 times, allowing vibrations to deeply penetrate your mind and body.

Kapalabhati (Skull Shining Breath)

This vigorous technique invigorates the mind and body, cleansing the nasal passages and lungs and boosting the digestive system's fire.

1. Sit in a comfortable position with your spine straight.
2. Take a deep breath, and as you exhale, pull your stomach in sharply, forcing the breath out in a short burst.
3. Let your inhalation be passive, with your focus on the forceful exhalations.
4. Continue this pattern of short, forceful exhales and passive inhales. Aim for a steady, rhythmic pace. Beginners can start with one exhale per second, gradually increasing speed as they become more comfortable.
5. Perform 30 such breaths to complete one round. Rest, then perform two more rounds.

Sitali Breath (Cooling Breath)

Sitali helps to cool the body, calm the mind, and soothe the nervous system.

1. Sit in a comfortable position with your eyes closed.
2. Curl the sides of your tongue upward into a tube (if you're unable to curl your tongue, you can purse your lips slightly instead).
3. Inhale through the tongue or lips, and feel the cooling sensation as the air passes.

4. Close your mouth and exhale through your nose.
5. Repeat 5-10 times, focusing on the cooling sensation that spreads throughout your body.

Tummo Breathing (Inner Fire Breath)

Often used in Tibetan meditation practices, Tummo breathing helps ignite internal heat and awaken spiritual energy.

1. Sit with your back straight and relax your shoulders.
2. Inhale deeply through your nose, filling your lungs completely.
3. Hold your breath and contract your abdominal and pelvic muscles, directing energy toward your chest.
4. Exhale slowly through your nose as you relax the contractions and feel the warmth spread throughout your body.
5. Repeat several times, focusing on the rising internal heat with each cycle.

Integrating Pranayama with Meditation

Combining pranayama with meditation enhances the benefits of both practices, creating a powerful tool for deepening relaxation and improving mental clarity. After performing a pranayama technique, transition smoothly into meditation by sitting quietly, observing the changes in your breath, and allowing your mind to achieve a state of stillness. This combination helps achieve a higher state of awareness and stabilizes the mind and body, promoting a profound sense of inner peace and balance.

TESTIMONIES OF TRANSFORMATION

Breathwork and pranayama, ancient disciplines rooted in rhythmic control and breath awareness, have shown remarkable efficacy in treating conditions linked to low vagal tone, such as anxiety disorders and cardiovascular issues. These personal stories highlight the transformative power of these practices.

Darius's Revival with Diaphragmatic Breathing: Darius, a 45-year-old small business owner, struggled with asthma and chronic bronchitis. Constantly battling shortness of breath and persistent coughing, he began incorporating diaphragmatic breathing into his daily routine. This simple practice led to significant improvements in his respiratory health, increasing lung volume, reducing breathlessness and chronic cough. Enhanced oxygen flow improved his mental clarity and energy levels, allowing Darius to manage his symptoms effectively and regain control over his life.

Gabriela's Calm through Resonant Breathing: Gabriela, a 36-year-old performing artist, struggled with phobias and a pervasive sense of insecurity that affected her stage presence. By practicing resonant breathing, she found calm and balance before performances. Over time, Gabriela's confidence grew, positively impacting her performances and overall sense of security.

Raj's Relief with Nadi Shodhana: Raj, a 33-year-old doctor, was under constant pressure, suffering from chronic stress and tension headaches. He incorporated Nadi Shodhana, or alternate nostril breathing, into his daily routine. This technique helped him balance his nervous system, reducing stress and alleviating his headaches. Practicing Nadi Shodhana before and after his shifts significantly improved Raj's resilience and ability to handle his demanding job.

Numerous studies support the clinical benefits of these breathing techniques. Research published in the *Journal of Clinical Psychology* demonstrated that individuals with chronic anxiety showed significant reductions in anxiety scores after an 8-week course of structured breathwork therapy. Another study on heart health revealed that patients who practiced daily pranayama and breathwork exercises had better heart rate variability and fewer symptoms of heart disease.

These testimonies and studies underscore the healing power of breathwork and its profound impact on mental and physical health, particularly through enhancing vagal tone. They serve as a reminder that true health often comes from within, from tuning into our body's natural rhythms. Let these insights inspire you to incorporate these practices into your daily routine, leading to a more balanced and healthy life.

CHAPTER 12
MINDFULNESS AND
MEDITATION

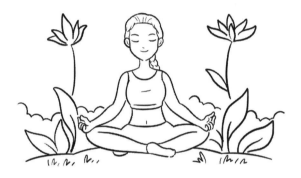

I n our fast-paced world, finding moments of stillness can be transformative. Meditation and mindfulness offer a powerful way to connect deeply with yourself. These techniques engage your mind and body in a harmonious dance that nurtures inner peace. This serene mental space allows your vagus nerve to function optimally, enhancing its tone and building resilience against daily stress. These practices are the access point to cultivate a calm, balanced life grounded in the present moment.

MINDFULNESS AND MEDITATION: SOOTHING THE VAGUS NERVE

Mindfulness involves maintaining a moment-by-moment awareness of our thoughts, feelings, bodily sensations, and the surrounding environment with openness, curiosity, and acceptance. Imagine an experience where every signal and sensation is acknowledged but not judged. When you engage in mindfulness, especially through meditation, you're training your brain to become more attuned to your body and environment, enhancing the tone of your vagus nerve.

Meditation, a cornerstone of mindfulness practice, involves focusing the mind on a particular object, thought, or activity to train attention and awareness. This practice induces relaxation and mental clarity, activating the vagus nerve and promoting a cascade of beneficial physiological changes.

The vagus nerve plays a vital role in regulating heart rate, controlling muscle movement, and sending anti-inflammatory signals throughout the body. When you meditate, focusing on your breath or the sensations in your body, you activate this nerve, promoting a state of calm and relaxation and enhancing your body's resilience to stressors. This physiological transformation highlights the power of mindful practices.

Studies have shown that neurobiologically, regular engagement in mindfulness and meditation increases gray matter density in the brain, particularly in areas associated with emotional regulation, such as the prefrontal cortex and hippocampus. These changes enhance cognitive functions and reduce activity in the amygdala, the brain's fear center, which is heavily involved in processing stress and anxiety. This neuroplasticity—the brain's ability to reorganize itself by forming new neural connections—demonstrates the profound impact of mindfulness on the brain's structure and function.

Research findings have consistently demonstrated that mindfulness meditation is associated with improvements in heart rate variability (HRV), a direct marker of vagal tone. For instance, a study published in the journal 'Psychoneuroendocrinology' found that individuals who engaged in an eight-week mindfulness-based stress reduction program showed significant increases in HRV, indicating enhanced vagal modulation of heart rate. These improvements were linked to reduced anxiety and depression symptoms, highlighting the therapeutic potential of mindfulness in regulating emotional health through vagal pathways.

Techniques and Practices

To begin your practice, you might explore guided mindfulness meditation focusing on breath and body sensations. Here's how you can start:

- Find a quiet, comfortable place to sit or lie down.
- Close your eyes and take a few deep breaths to center yourself.
- Shift your attention to your natural breathing pattern without trying to change it. Notice the sensation of air entering and leaving your nostrils.
- As you settle into the rhythm of your breath, expand your awareness to include the sensations in your

body. Feel the weight of your body against the chair or floor.

- If your mind wanders, gently acknowledge the thoughts and return your focus to your breath or body sensations.

For those who find sitting still challenging, don't worry—other effective practices exist. Guided imagery and progressive muscle relaxation also stimulate the vagus nerve. These techniques release physical tension and promote deep relaxation. You can read more about these methods in another section of the book.

Consistency is the key to getting the full benefits of mindfulness and meditation. Like a musician who practices daily to master their instrument, you must regularly engage with mindfulness to tune your vagus nerve. Over time, this consistent practice can significantly improve your physical and emotional well-being. Think of mindfulness as a cornerstone of holistic health—regular practice helps solidify its positive effects.

Even a few minutes daily can make a difference if you're just starting. Try setting aside a specific time each day for your practice, whether in the morning to set a calm tone for the day or in the evening to wind down. The important thing is to make it a regular part of your routine. Consistency helps you build a habit; soon, mindfulness will become a natural and beneficial part of your everyday life.

EMOTIONAL FREEDOM TECHNIQUE: TAPPING INTO THE BENEFITS OF MODERN ACUPRESSURE

In the tapestry of holistic healing practices, the Emotional Freedom Technique (EFT), often called "tapping," emerges as a fascinating thread. EFT combines the ancient wisdom of acupressure with modern understanding of the body's energy meridians, making it accessible, empowering, and highly effective. At its heart, EFT is a self-administered healing technique involving rhythmic tapping on specific body points, known as meridian points. These points, used in traditional Chinese medicine for acupuncture, are believed to be energy flow vortexes throughout the body.

The beauty of EFT lies in its simplicity and the profound theory it rests upon—that emotional distress and many physical ailments result from disruptions in the body's energy system. By tapping on these meridian points while focusing on specific negative emotions or physical sensations, EFT releases energy flow blockages, restores balance, and promotes emotional and physical healing. This practice aligns closely with the functions of the vagus nerve, which acts as a bridge between the brain and the body's internal organs, regulating relaxation responses and helping manage stress reactions.

The efficacy of EFT extends beyond anecdotal success stories; a growing body of scientific research backs it. Studies have shown that tapping can significantly decrease psychological stress markers, reduce anxiety, and improve mood. Notably, a review published in the "Journal of Nervous and Mental Disease" found that EFT helps reduce anxiety scores among people with anxiety disorders. Furthermore, its benefits are not just immediate; they can also be long-lasting, providing an effective tool for emotional regulation and stress management.

Guided EFT Exercises

The practice may seem unusual for those new to EFT, yet its techniques are straightforward and quick to learn. Here are a few basic routines to get you started:

The Basic Recipe:

1. Identify an issue you wish to focus on and rate the intensity of your feeling or discomfort on a scale from 0 to 10.
2. Tap on the "karate chop" point (the soft part of the hand below the pinkie and above the wrist) while reciting a setup statement acknowledging the issue and affirming self-acceptance, such as, "Even though I have this [anxiety], I deeply and completely accept myself."
3. Tap about seven times each on the following points while focusing on your emotion: eyebrow, side of the eye, under the eye, under the nose, chin, beginning of the collarbone, and under the arm.

The Calming Sequence: For moments of acute stress or anxiety:

1. Start tapping on the side of the hand and progress to the top of the head, eyebrow, side of the eye, under the eye, nose, chin, and collarbone.
2. With each tap, breathe deeply and focus on a mantra like, "I am calm and in control."

The Quick Anxiety Relief: If you feel a sudden onset of anxiety:

1. Tap continuously on the under-eye point while taking deep, slow breaths.
2. Think about the stressor and mentally reassure yourself, "I am safe now."

Incorporating EFT into Everyday Life

One advantage of EFT is its versatility and ease of integration into daily routines. You can use EFT in almost any setting without special tools or privacy. For instance, while waiting in line or traffic, you can discreetly tap on the side of your hand or under the arm to manage rising feelings of impatience or stress. After a challenging meeting or during a break at work, a few minutes spent tapping can reset your emotional state, reducing feelings of overwhelm and restoring focus.

EFT is a testament to the power of integrating ancient healing traditions with contemporary therapeutic practices. It offers a practical, accessible means of fostering emotional and physical health that honors the complex interconnections of our minds and bodies. As you explore and apply the techniques of EFT, you may find it an invaluable ally in your quest for wellness.

GUIDED VISUALIZATION FOR VAGAL TONE IMPROVEMENT

In the landscape of your mind, where thoughts often run wild like untamed winds, visualization is a potent tool that can transform these breezes into a gentle, rhythmic flow that nurtures your body and soul. When you visualize, you're not merely daydreaming but creating an inner sanctuary that can influence your body's most intricate systems.

Visualization operates on the principle that your mind can affect your body's biology. When you engage in this practice, you send signals to your brain to interpret it as real, sensory experiences. These signals can initiate a cascade of physical responses, particularly activating the vagus nerve, which mediates between your emotional and physiological states. By guiding your mind through specific, positive scenarios, you can elicit a relaxation response in your body, mediated by the vagus nerve. This response helps reduce stress, lower heart rate, decrease blood pressure, and promote overall well-being.

Simple Visualization Exercises

To harness the benefits of guided visualization, here are three simple exercises designed to stimulate your vagus nerve and enhance your vagal tone:

- **The Forest Path**: Close your eyes and imagine yourself strolling through a lush, green forest. The sun peeks through the leaves, casting warm, dappled light across the path. With each step, feel the soft earth under your feet, hear the gentle rustling of leaves, and breathe in the fresh, pine-scented air. As you walk, imagine a sense of calm spreading through your body, from the crown of your head to the tips of your toes. Each breath brings deeper relaxation, engaging your vagus nerve and soothing your entire body.

- **Ocean Waves**: Picture yourself sitting on a peaceful beach as the sun sets in vibrant hues of orange and pink. In front of you, the ocean waves gently lap against the shore. Visualize the rhythmic pattern of the waves: inhale as the wave pulls away from the beach, and exhale as it rolls back in. Sync your breathing with this ebb and flow, allowing the steady rhythm to calm your mind and activate your vagus nerve, enhancing your body's relaxation response.

- **Healing Light**: Imagine a beam of soothing, warm light shining down from above, bathing you in its radiance. See this light as a healing force, moving slowly over your body, beginning at your head and gradually working its way down to your feet. As this light touches each part of your body, feel it relaxing and healing, releasing any tension or discomfort. Focus on the sensation of warmth and light, expanding your chest area each time you breathe in, stimulating your vagus nerve, and promoting a deep sense of peace throughout your body.

Incorporating into Daily Routine

Integrating guided visualization into your daily routine can amplify its benefits, making it a powerful tool in your wellness arsenal. Consider setting aside a few minutes each morning or evening to practice visualization. It can be as simple as spending five minutes before you start your day or unwinding before bed. You can also use visualization techniques during breaks throughout the day to reset your stress levels and boost your mood.

TESTIMONIES OF TRANSFORMATION

Mindfulness and meditation are potent tools for stress management, chronic pain alleviation, and emotional resilience. Here are inspiring stories of individuals who transformed their lives through these practices.

Olivia's Relief through Mindfulness Meditation Olivia, a 30-year-old teacher managing fibromyalgia and chronic pain, found significant relief through mindfulness meditation. Dedicating just 15 minutes each morning to her practice, Olivia experienced a noticeable decrease in her pain levels and mood. This allowed her to engage more fully with her students and her personal life, transforming her daily experience.

Tasha's Comfort with EFT Tasha, a 49-year-old X-ray technician with a compromised immune system due to cancer treatment, lived in constant fear for her future. Desperate for relief, she discovered the Emotional Freedom Technique (EFT). By tapping on specific meridian points while acknowledging her fears, she experienced a profound shift to accept her situation, creating a calmer, state of mind, positively impacting her immune response. Her treatments were more effective and the frequency of infections diminished, giving her renewed hope.

Sofia's Serenity through Visualization At 41, media producer Sofia struggled with debilitating panic attacks and incessant worry. She embraced visualization techniques to combat her anxiety, picturing tranquil walks through forested paths. This daily practice not only stabilized her emotions but also brought her physiological responses under control—her heart rate slowed, instilling a deep calm. Empowered by this newfound peace, Sofia navigated her high-pressure job with renewed confidence and poise.

Research firmly supports the power of mindfulness to enhance vagal tone, with studies demonstrating that regular practice can significantly boost heart rate variability (HRV), a critical measure of vagal health. For instance, a study in Psychosomatic Medicine revealed that participants in an 8-week mindfulness-based stress reduction (MBSR) program not only saw increased HRV but also experienced notable reductions in stress, highlighting the profound benefits of engaging the mind-body connection. These findings, alongside inspiring personal stories, underscore how mindfulness and meditation are more than just therapeutic tools—they are gateways to a lifestyle marked by reduced stress, heightened mental clarity, and deeper inner connections. By adopting these practices, you are not just easing symptoms but fostering a resilient, peaceful, and holistically healthy life.

CHAPTER 13
SOUND AND VIBRATION TECHNIQUES

The gentle hum of a soothing melody or the resonant tone of a singing bowl are more than just soothing sounds; they are gateways to profound healing. This chapter explores the fascinating interplay between sound, vibration, and the vagus nerve. Here, you will discover how specific sounds and frequencies activate deep, visceral responses that promote healing and well-being.

SOUND THERAPY AND THE VAGUS NERVE: HEALING FREQUENCIES

Sound therapy, an ancient art revitalized by modern science, taps into the natural rhythms and frequencies that resonate with our bodies at a cellular level. At the heart of sound therapy is that all matter, including the human body, vibrates at specific frequencies. When these natural frequencies become disrupted—by stress, illness, or environmental factors—sound therapy can help realign them, fostering health and harmony.

The importance of sound and vibration healing lies in its ability to tap into the body's inherent capacity for self-regulation and healing. Our bodies, composed of approximately 70% water, are highly receptive to sound vibrations. These vibrations can penetrate cells and tissues, promoting balance and alignment at a cellular level. When the body's natural frequencies become disrupted due to stress, illness, or environmental factors, sound therapy helps realign them, fostering a state of harmony and well-being. This approach not only addresses the symptoms but also the root causes of various health issues, making it a holistic and non-invasive form of therapy.

Scientific research supports the efficacy of sound and vibration healing in improving health outcomes. For example, a study published in the Journal of Evidence-Based Complementary & Alternative Medicine found that participants who listened to sound frequencies in the range of 528 Hz experienced significant reductions in stress and anxiety levels, as this frequency is often associated with DNA repair and relaxation effects. Another study in the Journal of Advanced Nursing demonstrated that patients exposed to music therapy, including frequencies around 60-70 beats per minute (which mimics the resting heart rate), had lower blood pressure and heart rate, indicating a direct impact on the autonomic nervous system.

The vagus nerve is particularly receptive to and influenced by sound. It responds to auditory stimuli by modulating heart rate, respiratory rate, and digestive functions. For instance, calming music or the rhythmic tone of a singing bowl can trigger the release of acetylcholine, a neurotransmitter that lowers heart rate and promotes relaxation. This is a form of neural therapy that can manage stress, anxiety, and other conditions by enhancing vagal tone and improve your body's ability to relax and heal.

Sound and vibration healing harness the body's natural frequencies to promote health and wellness to address both physical and emotional imbalances through non-invasive means. Sound therapy offers a promising and accessible way to enhance the body's natural healing processes, making it a valuable addition to modern therapeutic practices and a very simple way to tap into one of the most fundamental aspects of your own biology.

BINAURAL BEATS AND NEUROMODULATION

Picture yourself in a quiet space, wearing headphones, as a wave of audio tones washes over you. Each ear hears tones of slightly different frequencies, creating a third, perceived tone in the brain, a binaural beat. This form of soundwave therapy operates on a simple principle: the unique sound waves encourage your brain to sync its wave frequencies with this new 'beat.' This alignment can lead to mental states that promote healing, relaxation, and improved mental health.

The interaction between binaural beats and the vagus nerve is particularly fascinating. This nerve, responsible for regulating the body's relaxation response, can be stimulated by specific auditory frequencies provided by binaural beats. Listening to these beats encourages your brain to produce brainwave patterns associated with relaxation and meditation. For example, when you set the difference in frequency between the tones in each ear to promote theta wave production, which links to deep relaxation and meditation, you stimulate the vagus nerve to enhance its tone. This increased vagal tone can lead to a reduced heart rate, lower blood pressure, and a feeling of calm, effectively reducing stress and anxiety.

The implications of this for mental health are profound. Various studies have shown that binaural beats can help manage symptoms of anxiety, stress, and even insomnia. By inducing brainwaves that promote relaxation, these beats can help interrupt the feedback loop of anxiety, where the brain gets stuck in a state of heightened alertness. For individuals struggling with sleep, the right frequency can coax the brain into producing waves that naturally occur at the onset of sleep, helping combat insomnia without medication.

For optimal results, the use of binaural beats should follow specific guidelines. First, you must use headphones because binaural beats rely on delivering two slightly different tones into each ear to create the perception of a third tone. You can vary the duration and frequency of listening depending on your needs and the conditions you are addressing. Starting with shorter sessions and gradually increasing the duration can help your brain adjust to and integrate the experience more effectively. Typically, sessions can range from 15 to 30 minutes. Choosing recordings tuned to frequencies that promote the desired mental states is also crucial as different frequencies can elicit relaxation, sleep, or heightened focus.

By exploring the potential of binaural beats and under-standing their ability to modulate brainwave activity and stimulate the vagus nerve, you can tap into a profound tool for mental and physical health. It's a testament to the incredible adaptability of our brains and ongoing innovation in the field of neuromodulation, offering new avenues for healing and well-being. As we continue to uncover the intricate connections between sound, brainwaves, and bodily health, binaural beats stand out as a promising area of exploration, blending the ancient with the modern in the ongoing journey toward holistic health.

OUR OWN POWERFUL VIBRATIONS: YOUR VOICEBOX HEALS

In the symphony of healing techniques that engage the vagus nerve, your own voice plays a pivotal role that often goes unnoticed. It's not just about your words but how you use your voice through humming, singing, gargling, and chanting. These activities stimulate your vagus nerve, promoting relaxation and enhancing your body's natural healing abilities. The science of vibration underpins this interaction, where specific vocal tones and frequencies resonate to trigger a vagus nerve response, leading to improved mood, decreased stress, and better respiratory health.

Think of your body as an instrument, with your vocal apparatus vibrating like the strings on a guitar to produce sound. Vocal activities such as humming, singing, gargling, and chanting generate vibrations that stimulate the vagus nerve, particularly around the throat and chest. This stimulation can increase heart rate variability—a marker of a healthy nervous system—and lower stress levels by triggering the release of relaxation-inducing neurotransmitters. Humming calms the mind and resonates in the head and neck, directly stimulating the vagus nerve. Singing, whether casually or in church or choir groups, provides these same benefits but also enhances mood. Gargling activates the muscles in the back of the throat sending vibrations deep within the body.Chanting aligns breath and voice, often used in meditation to enhance focus and reduce stress, and its vibrations stimulate the vagus nerve.

Integrating these voice therapies into your daily routine can be seamless and with little to no disruption. Consider humming your favorite tune while preparing breakfast, doing laundry, or singing in your car on your morning commute. These activities not only uplift your spirit during mundane tasks but also bring therapeutic benefits of vagal stimulation. Similarly, you can incorporate gargling into your morning and nighttime bathroom routines, ensuring regular vagus nerve stimulation.

Chanting can be particularly effective while engaging in gardening or gentle stretching activities. Here are a few simple chants that you can start with:

- **Om**: Often used in meditation, repeating the sound 'Om' can help calm the mind and reduce stress. Find a comfortable seated position. Take a deep breath through your nose. As you exhale, chant "OM" with a prolonged and steady sound, starting with "A," moving through "U," and ending with "M." Feel the vibration of the sound resonating throughout your body. Repeat several times, focusing on the sound and its calming effect.

- **Sa Ta Na Ma**: A Kundalini yoga mantra, this chant promotes mental balance and well-being. Find a comfortable seated position with your spine straight. Close your eyes and take a few deep breaths to relax your mind and body. **Sa:** Touch the index finger to the thumb and chant "Sa" (pronounced like "suh") as you pull the navel point in rhythmically. **Ta:** Touch the middle finger to the thumb and chant "Ta" (pronounced like "tuh") as you press the navel point in. **Na:** Touch the ring finger to the thumb and chant "Na" (pronounced like "nah") as you release the navel point out. **Ma:** Touch the little finger to the thumb and chant "Ma" (pronounced like "mah") as you press the navel point in. Continue chanting "Sa Ta Na Ma" in a steady rhythm, coordinating the movements of your fingers with the sounds and the navel point. Reflect on the meaning of the mantra, which represents the cycle of life, death, rebirth, and the transformational process. After chanting for a desired duration, take a few moments to sit quietly and feel the effects of the mantra on your mind and body.
- **Ho'oponopono Prayer**: This Hawaiian prayer—"I'm sorry, Please forgive me, Thank you, I love you"—is a powerful, repetitive chant that unlocks emotional blocks and fosters forgiveness and positive energy. You can play many musical variations while chanting or simply repeat the statements repeatedly in a meditative format.

Integrating these practices into your life can significantly enhance your well-being by leveraging the healing power of your voice.

TESTIMONIES OF TRANSFORMATION

Sound and vibration techniques harness the power of auditory and vibrational stimuli to promote healing, reduce stress, and enhance well-being. These inspiring stories highlight the transformative impact of these practices.

Colton's Calm through Binaural Beats: Colton, a 40-year-old creative director, was overwhelmed by chronic stress and debilitating tension headaches. Seeking relief, he turned to binaural beats. This therapy allowed Colton to process and release the physical manifestations of stress stored in his body. The result was not only a dramatic reduction in his headaches but also a surge in creative energy and productivity. Colton's newfound vitality transformed his professional and personal life, showcasing the profound impact of somatic therapy.

Mei's Peace through Humming: Mei, a 28-year-old designer plagued by insomnia and intrusive thoughts, discovered the soothing power of humming. She incorporated humming into her nightly routine, using it as a meditative practice while tidying her apartment and taking her evening shower. This simple technique quieted her mind before bed, improving her sleep quality and reducing intrusive thoughts. Mei's overall well-being significantly improved, showcasing the profound impact of such a simple practice.

Omar's Balance with Chanting and Singing: Omar, a 52-year-old therapist managing diabetes and obesity, struggled with being present for his patients and feeling comfortable in his own skin. Starting with just five minutes of chanting in the shower, Omar noticed a dramatic improvement in his focus at work. Inspired, he began alternating between chanting and singing during his commute. The repetitive vocalization of soothing mantras reduced his stress and enhanced his focus, while singing brought him joy and connected him with his body. Over time, Omar experienced improvements in his mental clarity and emotional balance, positively impacting his health and professional practice.

As you explore these vocal techniques, remember that consistency is key. Regularly integrating these practices into your life, rather than focusing on intensity, will yield the most benefits. By doing so, you're not just singing or humming; you're activating your body's natural healing abilities and nurturing your overall well-being.

In embracing the power of your voice, you tap into a simple yet profound tool for health and healing. As we conclude this exploration of sound and vibration techniques, remember that these methods are not just about engaging with sound— they are about engaging with yourself on a deeper level. Tune into your body's needs, actively participate in your journey to wellness, and recognize the accessible and powerful tools you possess. This chapter encourages you to use these tools to their fullest potential, fostering a healthier and more harmonious life.

HELP SPREAD THE WORD

"In our willingness to give that which we seek, we keep the abundance of the universe circulating in our lives."

DEEPAK CHOPRA

Dear Reader,

Thank you for picking up this book. Writing it has been a crucial part of my healing journey, and I'm so grateful to share it with you and be part of your journey too.

To keep the positive feedback loop Deepak Chopra mentions and circulate abundance in both our lives and the lives of others, you can help this book get in front of the people that need it most by writing an honest review.

Scan the QR code to leave your review.

Use the simple techniques and exercises in the coming chapters to dig in on your journey to wellness.

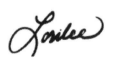

CHAPTER 14

MOVEMENT AND PHYSICAL EXERCISES

Your body is a dynamic landscape where each movement shapes the terrain and each breath alters the atmosphere. Movement can be a powerful tool for stimulating the vagus nerve, enhancing your parasympathetic tone and promoting a cascade of health benefits that ripple through every aspect of your well-being. This chapter delves into various physical exercises and explains how you can harness them to activate the vagus nerve, fostering a state of calm and balance.

YOGA AND THE VAGUS NERVE: ASANAS FOR ACTIVATION

With its ancient roots and modern adaptations, yoga offers more than just physical benefits; it is a therapeutic power-house for your vagus nerve. The magic of yoga lies in its ability to transform your physiological state. When you practice yoga, you are not just moving your body; you send signals along the vagus nerve that calm your heart rate, regulate your digestive functions, and decrease your stress levels. Each pose and each breath acts like a message of tranquility, enhancing your body's parasympathetic responses.The following yoga poses are particularly effective in activating the vagus nerve:

Uttanasana (Standing Forward Bend)

Calms the nervous system, promotes deep diaphragmatic breathing, stimulates the vagus nerve, reduces stress, and enhances relaxation. From standing, inhale deeply as you raise your arms above your head, and as you exhale, hinge at your hips and fold forward, bringing your chest towards your thighs. Allow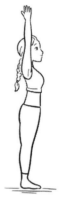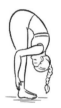
your head to hang heavy, and reach your hands towards the floor, ankles, or shins. Keep a slight bend in your knees if necessary to avoid straining your lower back.

Setu Bandhasana (Bridge Pose)

Strengthens the back while opening up the chest and lungs, enhancing breathing and activating the vagus nerve. Lie on your back with knees bent and feet flat on the floor, lift your hips towards the ceiling.

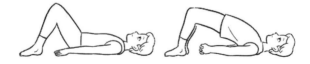

Balasana (Child's Pose)

This forward bending posture facilitates a sense of safety and comfort—a haven for your nervous system. Kneel on the floor, hip width apart or wider, sit back on your heels, and stretch your arms forward, bringing your forehead to the floor.

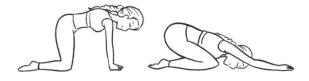

Marjaryasana-Bitilasana (Cat-Cow Pose)

The rhythmic, flowing movement of the Cat-Cow Pose increases spinal fluid circulation and gently massages the organs, stimulating the vagus nerve. This dynamic sequence involves alternating between Cat Pose (round the spine) and Cow Pose (arch the back).

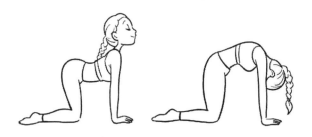

Viparita Karani (Legs Up the Wall Pose)

Promotes relaxation, reduces stress, and enhances circulation. The inversion helps calm the nervous system and stimulate the vagus nerve. Lie on your back with your legs extended up against a wall.

Savasana (Corpse Pose)

Promotes complete relaxation, reduces stress, and enhances the parasympathetic response, stimulating the vagus nerve. Lie flat on your back with your arms at your sides, palms facing up, and feet relaxed.

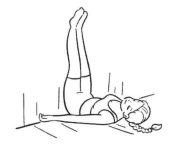

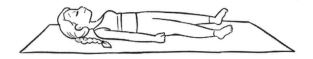

Integration with Mindful Breathing

Integrating mindful breathing with yoga poses is essential to maximize vagal activation. Techniques like Ujjayi Pranayama (Ocean Breath), where you constrict the back of your throat to create a gentle sound as you breathe, not only supports the physical execution of poses but also brings a meditative quality to your practice, helping to reduce mental noise and soothe the nervous system. Refer back to Chapter 11 for more breathwork ideas to integrate into your practice.

Engaging in yoga regularly offers a pathway to enhance physical flexibility and strength while fostering a deeper connection with your inner self. To gain the benefits, incorporate at least three poses daily, holding each for 3-5 minutes. As you incorporate these practices into your life, you may find a profound sense of harmony and health unfolding—a true testament to the power of integrating movement with mindful breathing.

GENTLE MOVEMENT AND PHYSICAL EXERCISES FOR VAGAL STIMULATION

Sometimes, gentle approaches are the most powerful for healing and self-care. Tai Chi and Chi Gong, with their slow, deliberate movements, enhance vagal tone and promote relaxation. Rooted in ancient traditions, they balance energy flow and ease the body into healing. Imagine slow fluidity to the movements as you visualize these options.

Tai Chi: Meditation in Motion

Tai Chi, often described as meditation in motion, involves a series of slow, focused movements accompanied by deep breathing. Each posture flows into the next without pause, ensuring your body is in constant motion.

- **Wave Hands like Clouds:** Stand with your feet shoulder-width apart, knees slightly bent, and gently wave your arms horizontally in front of you, mimicking the slow drift of clouds. This movement helps regulate your breathing and focus your mind, stimulating the vagus nerve and enhancing your parasympathetic response.
- **Brush Knee and Step Forward:** Step forward with one foot while sweeping your arms in a brush

motion. This motion helps in coordination and balance and calms your nervous system.

Chi Gong: Harnessing Energy Flow

Like Tai Chi, Chi Gong focuses on routines that align and calm the body, mind, and spirit through rhythm and gentle movements.

- **Swimming Dragon**: Begin by standing with your feet shoulder-width apart, knees slightly bent, and arms relaxed at your sides. Extend your arms forward, palms facing down, and slowly move them in a wave-like motion from side to side, allowing your torso and hips to follow the movement. As your arms and torso move, gently twist your spine, letting your hips sway naturally, imagining your body moving like a dragon swimming through water. Coordinate your breath with the movement, inhaling as you move to one side and exhaling as you move to the other. Continue this flowing, wave-like motion for 5-10 minutes, focusing on the gentle spinal twist and synchronized breath.
- **Bouncing Ball**: Stand with your feet shoulder-width apart, knees slightly bent, and arms relaxed at your sides. Raise your arms in front of you as if holding a large ball, palms facing each other. As you inhale, lift the imaginary ball up to chest level, then exhale and press it down towards your abdomen, bending your knees slightly as you lower your arms. Create a gentle bouncing effect with your body, imagining the ball is

buoyant and springy. Maintain a rhythmic flow of movement and breath, inhaling as you lift the ball and exhaling as you press it down. Continue this bouncing motion for 5-10 minutes.

Dance: Rhythmic Joy for Vagal Health

Transitioning to a more dynamic form of movement, dance can be an enjoyable way to stimulate your vagus nerve. Dance incorporates rhythmic, full-body movements that enhance physical fitness, elevate your mood, and positively impact your nervous system's health. The rhythmic nature of dance movements, especially in styles like salsa or ballroom, can synchronize with your heart rhythms, promoting cardiovascular health and improving vagal tone. Integrating dance into your daily routine can be as simple as playing your favorite tunes for a few minutes each day and allowing your body to move freely without judgment. This spontaneous, joyous form of movement can liberate you from stress and activate the parasympathetic nervous system, providing a healthy, refreshing break from the routine stresses of life.

Therapeutic Shaking: Releasing Tension

Consider the practice of therapeutic shaking, a less intense form of Trauma Release Exercise (TRE). This method involves simple exercises that induce therapeutic tremors in the body, which are natural nervous system responses to release tension and trauma. Start by standing with your feet hip-width apart and simply allow your knees to shake gently, progressing to letting the tremors move up your legs and through your torso. These vibrations help calm the nervous system by releasing held tension and enhancing the function of the vagus nerve. Another gentle shaking exercise involves lying on your back with your legs raised and slightly bent at the knees; gently rock your legs from side to side, allowing the movement to create a soft shaking sensation through your body. This exercise soothes the nervous system and aids in digestive function, a direct benefit of stimulating the vagus nerve.

Walking and Light Cardiovascular Exercises

Incorporating walking and light cardiovascular exercises into your daily life is another supportive way to enhance your vagal tone. A brisk walk in the morning, integrated with periods of mindful breathing, can kickstart your day by activating your vagus nerve and boosting your mood and metabolism. For those who enjoy a bit of fun while exercising, using a mini-trampoline for gentle bouncing can be an excellent way to stimulate your body's mechanoreceptors, activating the vagus nerve. Light bouncing is enjoyable and beneficial for lymphatic drainage and cardiovascular health. Aim for short sessions; even a few minutes can be helpful, and try to incorporate it into your routine a few times a week.

Pilates: Precision and Control for Vagal Activation

Pilates emphasizes precise, controlled movements and mindful breathing, offering a comprehensive approach to engaging the vagus nerve. Through exercises focusing on core strength and flexibility, Pilates helps regulate autonomic nervous system function, enhancing physical and mental health. The coordination of movement and breath in Pilates, like in yoga, is vital for stimulating the vagus nerve and promoting relaxation. Try incorporating Pilates sessions into your weekly routine, focusing on techniques that encourage deep, diaphragmatic breathing and core engagement, which are particularly effective for vagal stimulation.

Each of these practices provides unique benefits for your nervous system health, from the meditative movements of Tai Chi and Chi Gong to the joyful expression of dance and the precision of Pilates. They offer accessible, enjoyable ways to integrate physical activity into your life, enhancing your vagal tone and overall well-being. As you explore these options, remember that the key is consistency and mindfulness—by regularly engaging in these activities, you're not just moving your body; you're enhancing your life, one breath, one step, one dance at a time.

TESTIMONIES OF TRANSFORMATION

Movement therapies can be profoundly transformative, offering physical relief and emotional stability by engaging the vagus nerve and promoting a balanced nervous system. These stories of individuals who found healing through these practices highlight the powerful impact of movement on overall well-being.

Malik's Transformation with Yoga Asanas

Malik, a 55-year-old electrician struggling with chronic pain and depression, initially turned to yoga for gentle stretches to relieve his tight back muscles. Unexpectedly, he was introduced to breathwork during yoga. The combination of physical postures and mindful breathing helped him manage his pain and elevate his mood. Yoga became a transformative practice, providing both physical relief and emotional stability. It became a vital part of his weekly routine, something he eagerly anticipated.

Dakota's Calm through Tai Chi: Dakota, a 24-year-old university student experiencing tachycardia and extreme anxiety, found profound benefits in Tai Chi. She initially signed up to fulfill a GE requirement but soon discovered its deeper impact. With the slow, flowing movements, her persistent anxiety began to lift. This change wasn't temporary but lasting. Clinical assessments showed significant improvements in her heart rate variability (HRV), indicating enhanced vagal tone. The slow, deliberate movements and focused breathing helped regulate her heart rate and calm her mind. Regular Tai Chi practice reduced Dakota's anxiety episodes, allowing her to focus better on her studies and daily activities.

Layla's Reovery with Therapeutic Shaking: Layla, a 34-year-old nurse struggling with addiction to alcohol and drugs, was desperate for a way to manage her recovery. She discovered therapeutic shaking, a practice that helped her release pent-up tension and emotional stress. This outlet to experience and release emotion helped her to avoid numbing her emotions with drugs or alcohol. By regularly engaging in therapeutic shaking, Layla felt empowered and hopeful for long term recovery and was better equipped ot handle the daily stressors of her intense role helping others.

Group Study: Elderly Participants and Light Cardiovascular Exercise

A group study involving elderly participants engaged in daily light cardiovascular exercises such as walking and gentle aerobics. Over several months, their physical health improved, and they reported feeling happier and more connected. They also showed significant reductions in inflammation markers and improvements in HRV, highlighting the broader implications of light exercises for fostering community and improving quality of life among older adults.

These stories collectively paint a picture of how movement therapies can transform lives through vagal activation. They provide a blueprint for wellness that integrates body, mind, and spirit. For anyone on the path to recovery or seeking a more balanced life, these therapies offer gentle yet powerful tools for rejuvenation and healing. Embrace these practices and unlock the full potential of your body's natural healing abilities.

CHAPTER 15

SOMATIC AND SENSORY THERAPIES

SOMATIC EXPERIENCING: RELEASING TRAUMA THROUGH THE BODY

In the healing landscape, where each therapy offers a unique path to recovery, Somatic Experiencing (SE) stands out as a profound journey back to balance and health. This therapeutic approach, developed by Dr. Peter Levine, specifically eases trauma symptoms by engaging the body's innate ability to heal. It's a gentle yet powerful method that integrates the mind, emotions, and physiological responses, creating a sense of harmony many find elusive after traumatic experiences.

Somatic Experiencing is grounded in the observation that wild animals, though regularly threatened, rarely exhibit trauma symptoms. Their resilience stems from their unimpeded physical responses to threats, such as running or shaking, which effectively metabolize the high levels of stress energy triggered during a threat. Humans, however, often override these natural responses with rational behavior or social etiquette, leading to the entrapment of this survival energy in the nervous system. SE facilitates the completion of these pent-up survival responses, skillfully guiding you to tap into your body's wisdom, releasing trauma at a pace that feels safe and manageable.

Central to the process of Somatic Experiencing is the vagus nerve, a key component of your parasympathetic nervous system, often referred to as the 'rest and digest' system. In SE, the vagus nerve acts as a reset button to calm the nervous system after trauma disrupts its balance. SE practices restore the body's sense of safety, turning off the relentless 'threat' signals that keep the nervous system in a state of high alert. By doing so, these practices enhance the function of the vagus nerve, promoting a state of balance that supports recovery and resilience.

A typical Somatic Experiencing session is a collaboration in mindfulness, focusing on bodily sensations that arise as you recount or recall traumatic events. Instead of rehashing or reliving the trauma, which can be retraumatizing, SE works by noticing how your body reacts when discussing or remembering these events. You might notice sensations in your stomach, tightness in your chest, or clenching of your fists. Guided physical exercises encourage gentle exploration of these responses, which can involve simple movements, breathing exercises, or vocalizations promoting the release and regulation of trapped survival energies, facilitating a natural return to equilibrium.

Guided Somatic Exercises

Engaging in somatic exercises can dramatically shift your physiological state. For instance, if your muscles tighten as you recall a traumatic event, you might be guided to slowly and gently stretch or move that area. This movement can help release the bracing pattern your body has unconsciously adopted. Breathing techniques are also helpful; slow, deep, diaphragmatic breathing can stimulate the vagus nerve, encouraging a return to a calm state. These exercises are not just for sessions with a therapist; they can be integrated into your daily life, helping you to manage stress, reduce anxiety, and maintain a more balanced emotional state.

Somatic Experiencing offers a gentle path to healing for those who have felt stuck in their trauma responses. It acknowledges that trauma is not just a psychological issue but a physiological one that involves the entire body. By focusing on bodily sensations and the vagus nerve's role in regulating the body's response to stress, SE helps to release the grip of trauma, allowing for a return to profound and lasting wellness. As you continue to explore this and other somatic practices, remember that the journey to recovery is not just about reaching a destination but about rediscovering a life lived in balance and peace.

TRE: RELEASING TENSION AND TRAUMA THROUGH NEUROGENIC TREMORS

In the realm of therapeutic practices, TRE, or Tension and Trauma Releasing Exercises, pioneered by Dr. David Berceli, offer a unique approach to healing. This method utilizes the body's natural ability to release deep muscular tension and trauma patterns through induced shaking or tremoring. Initially, shaking may seem unusual—why shake intentionally? However, this process is deeply rooted in our biology; it's a primal recovery response that animals instinctively use in the wild after a threat has passed to restore their bodies to calm.

At its core, TRE, also called Neurogenic Tremoring or Therapeutic Shaking, is about safely activating this natural reflex to help the body let go of chronic stress or tension. The technique is grounded in the understanding that stress and trauma, whether physical or emotional, can lead to deep muscular tension that isn't always relieved through traditional forms of therapy. Over time, this unaddressed tension can manifest as mood disorders, chronic pain, and various other health issues. TRE addresses these deep-seated tensions, allowing the body to regain balance and relaxation.

The mechanism behind TRE involves a series of exercises that initially evoke voluntary muscle contractions, which then encourage the body to enter a state of involuntary tremoring. These tremors are generally mild and soothing, creating a wave-like sensation that travels through the body. This process fatigues the muscles and triggers a controlled shaking response, allowing the body to naturally release accumulated tension and restore the nervous system to equilibrium.

As you engage in TRE, this shaking mechanism profoundly influences the autonomic nervous system, which controls involuntary bodily functions, including heart rate, digestion, and respiratory rate. By initiating these neurogenic tremors, TRE helps shift the body from stress and alert (sympathetic dominance) to relaxation and recovery (parasympathetic dominance). This shift is crucial for enhancing vagal tone, as it stimulates the vagus nerve — your body's internal calm button — reducing stress hormones like cortisol and improving markers of resilience such as heart rate variability (HRV).

Guided TRE Exercises

To begin your TRE practice, you typically engage in simple, preparatory exercises that help mildly stress the muscles. Here are some steps to guide you:

1. **Ankle and Foot Stretch**: Stand and place your feet hip-width apart. Lift your heels off the ground and hold for a few seconds, then lower them. Repeat 5-10 times to activate the muscles in your legs.
2. **Knee Bends**: With feet hip-width apart, bend your knees slightly as if you're about to sit in a chair. Hold this position for a few seconds, then return to standing. Repeat 5-10 times to gently stress the thigh muscles.
3. **Wall Sit**: Lean against a wall and slide down until your thighs are parallel to the ground, as if sitting in an invisible chair. Hold this position for 1-2 minutes to engage the leg muscles fully.
4. **Lying on the Back**: After these preparatory exercises, lie down on your back with your knees bent and feet flat on the floor. Allow your knees to

fall towards each other, creating a relaxed position. This posture encourages the tremors to start naturally.

5. **Allowing the Tremors**: Relax and focus on your breath. As your body begins to tremor, let the shaking happen without trying to control or stop it. The tremors may start in the legs and move through the body. Allow the process to unfold naturally for 10-15 minutes.

Creating a Routine

Incorporating TRE into your wellness routine can be transformative, especially if done consistently. Practicing TRE two to three times a week provides significant benefits for most people. It's also highly synergistic with other practices that enhance vagal tone, such as deep breathing, yoga, or meditation. Combining TRE with these activities can amplify your body's relaxation response and accelerate your emotional and physical healing journey.

TRE represents a bridge to accessing your body's natural healing capabilities, providing a pathway to release, recover, and restore. As you explore this practice, remember that the journey is deeply personal and unique to each individual. Allow yourself the space and grace to explore TRE at your own pace, listening to your body's wisdom and respecting its limits as you learn to let go of the old tensions that no longer serve you.

EARTHING AND THE VAGUS NERVE: THE SCIENCE OF GROUNDING

When you consider the elements that affect well-being, the concept of earthing, or grounding, might not immediately spring to mind. Yet, this simple practice of connecting physically with the earth can profoundly affect your body, especially your nervous system and the vagus nerve. Earthing involves direct skin contact with the surface of the Earth, such as walking barefoot on grass, sand, or soil. The earth's surface has nearly a limitless supply of electrons that give it land, ocean and lakes a natural negative electric charge. When you connect to the earth, it dissipates static electricity and other environmental charges on you while simultaneously infusing your body with a charge of energy in the form of free electrons, synchronizing you to the natural frequencies of the earth.

Research supports the benefits of grounding, showing that this practice can help reduce chronic inflammatory and autoimmune diseases. It's believed that the electrons you absorb can help neutralize free radicals in your body, which are involved in inflammatory processes. A study published in the Journal of Inflammation Research noted significant improvements in inflammation and pain management among participants who practiced earthing. These findings are particularly relevant considering the vagus nerve's role in inflammation. By enhancing the body's response to inflammation, earthing can help stimulate the vagus nerve, reducing stress levels and inducing a state of calm. Physiologically, this shift manifests as reduced cortisol levels, decreased heart rate, and lower blood pressure, all regulated by the vagus nerve.

Additionally, improved heart rate variability, a key marker of vagal tone, has been observed with regular grounding practices, indicating enhanced resilience and stress management.

Practical Earthing Techniques

Incorporating earthing into your daily routine can be simple and practical, regardless of your living environment. Walking barefoot for about 30 minutes daily on grass, sand, or dirt can be immensely beneficial. If you live in an urban area, grounding mats or sheets can be used indoors to replicate the earth's electrical properties, proving helpful when used while sleeping, working, or relaxing at home.

For continuous grounding benefits, especially in social settings where removing your shoes is not feasible, consider using earthing footwear. These shoes, constructed with conductive materials, maintain a connection between your body and the earth throughout the day.

Technological advancements now allow you to enjoy the benefits of earthing even indoors. Earthing sheets and mats can be used in your home and office, especially beneficial for those living in high-rise buildings or climates where outdoor earthing is impractical year-round. These devices can be connected to the grounding wire in electrical outlets or directly to the earth via a wire, providing a continuous transfer of electrons to the body.

Whether walking barefoot outdoors or using indoor earthing techniques, connecting with the earth can significantly enhance your vagal tone and overall well-being. These practices are powerful tools in managing stress, reducing inflammation, and promoting a deep sense of calm. Integrating earthing into your wellness regimen offers a natural and accessible path to health and vitality.

SENSORY DEPRIVATION CHAMBERS: WATCH YOUR STRESS FLOAT AWAY

In the pursuit of tranquility and a reset for the nervous system, sensory deprivation chambers, also known as float tanks, provide a unique and profound way to stimulate the vagus nerve and induce deep relaxation and meditation. These tanks eliminate external sensory input, allowing you to drop into a state of profound calm. The principle relies on the idea that reducing sensory input to the brain naturally shifts focus inward, enhancing self-regulation and promoting a meditative state. This state activates the parasympathetic nervous system, which the vagus nerve significantly influences.

Essentially, float tanks are enclosed bathtubs, large enough to lie down in, filled with water saturated with Epsom salts. This high salt concentration allows you to float effortlessly. The water is heated to skin temperature, blurring the boundaries between the body and the water. With the tank completely soundproof and optionally darkened, it dramatically reduces the usual barrage of stimuli that flood your senses. This sensory reduction allows the vagus nerve to shift from managing external stimuli to enhancing internal balance and regeneration. The direct impact on the vagus nerve can lead to lower blood pressure, reduced heart rate, and decreased stress-related hormones, fostering an environment conducive to deep relaxation and healing.

The water in float tanks isn't just plain water; it's a solution rich in Epsom salts, which is magnesium sulfate. This salt solution is what keeps you buoyant, but that's not all. It is also absorbed through your skin, providing your body with magnesium, a 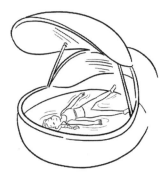 mineral essential for over 300 biochemical reactions. Magnesium is crucial in nerve function, muscle relaxation, and stress reduction. It helps regulate neurotransmitter systems directly linked to the vagus nerve, enhancing its ability to maintain calm and balance within your nervous system. This mineral's presence in the float tank water can help alleviate muscle tension and reduce physical stress, reinforcing the profound relaxation effects facilitated by the sensory deprivation experience.

Common Misperceptions and Fears

Floating in a sensory-deprived environment may initially seem intimidating, but common concerns like claustrophobia, boredom, or hygiene can be addressed and alleviated with proper information and preparation. Modern float tanks prioritize safety and comfort, featuring customizable settings that allow users to control light and sound according to their comfort level. For those uneasy about complete darkness or silence, starting with soft lighting and gentle music can ease the transition into sensory deprivation. Tanks are thoroughly filtered between each use, maintaining high standards of cleanliness and hygiene. By understanding these elements, you can confidently approach your first float, knowing you can tailor the experience to your comfort level.

TESTIMONIES OF TRIUMPH

Somatic and sensory therapies engage the body and senses to promote profound healing and well-being. By tapping into the body's natural responses and the power of sensory experiences, these methods can alleviate deep-seated tension, reduce stress, and enhance overall health. Here are some powerful stories that highlight the transformative impact of these approaches.

Christina's Recovery through Somatic Experiencing

Christina, a 48-year-old social worker, turned to Somatic Experiencing (SE) to recover from PTSD after a severe car accident. Each time she sat in a car, her heart raced and her breath quickened, symptoms of her trauma-induced hyperarousal state. Through SE, Christina learned to tune into these bodily sensations and work through them in real-time. Gradually, she began to feel calm while in a car, as her nervous system disengaged from its hyperarousal state. Her recovery was not just about reducing symptoms; it was about reclaiming her freedom to drive without fear.

Aisha's Strength with TRE

Aisha, a 37-year-old counselor, struggled with the lingering effects of sexual trauma and chronic muscle tension. She discovered Tension and Trauma Releasing Exercises (TRE), which enabled her to release deeply held physical and emotional tension. This practice led to significant improvements in her well-being. Aisha regained her strength and resilience, empowering her both personally and professionally. The liberation she felt from TRE was a testament to its power in healing deep-seated trauma.

Luis's Health Improvement through Earthing

Luis, a 50-year-old plumber dealing with hypertension, stumbled upon an unexpected remedy in earthing. One particularly hot day after work, he decided to unwind in the park with a cold drink. On a whim, he kicked off his boots and walked barefoot in the grass. The sensation was so soothing that he started making this a regular habit. Spending time barefoot in nature helped Luis connect with the Earth's natural energies, which lowered his blood pressure and reduced his stress levels. This simple yet powerful practice became a daily ritual for Luis, leading to significant health improvements and a calmer, more centered state of being.

Carlos' Respiratory Health with Float Tanks

Carlos, a 44-year-old mechanic, struggled with chronic constipation and high stress. Initially skeptical and fearful of the enclosed, sensory-deprived environment of float tanks, he decided to try it with options like dimmed lights and soft music for his first experience. To his surprise, the sessions provided deep relaxation and significant stress reduction. The buoyancy and sensory deprivation, along with the absorption of Epsom salt magnesium, improved his digestive health and resilience to stress. Over time, his chronic constipation eased, and he felt more capable of handling daily stressors. Float tanks became a sanctuary of calm for Carlos, significantly enhancing his overall well-being.

These testimonies illustrate the powerful and transformative effects of somatic and sensory therapies. By integrating these practices into their lives, individuals can unlock profound healing and well-being. These therapies offer more than just relief from symptoms—they provide a pathway to rejuvenation, resilience, and holistic health. Embrace these approaches and discover the incredible potential of engaging with your body's natural healing processes.

CHAPTER 16

BODYWORK AND TOUCH THERAPIES

BODYWORK FOR BALANCE: TAPPING INTO HEALING TOUCH AND ENERGETIC MODALITIES

Imagine your body as a complex network of highways where messages of both pain and healing are constantly transmitted. Now, imagine having the power to direct these messages, to shift the pathways from pain to relief, from dissonance to harmony. This power lies at your fingertips through the healing art of bodywork and touch therapies. In this chapter, we explore how touch therapies not only soothe the surface of your skin but also communicate with your body's internal network, particularly the vagus nerve, promoting healing and restoring balance.

Touch is more than just a sensory experience—it's a vital communication tool that can profoundly enhance your health. When your skin perceives touch, it sends signals directly to the vagus nerve through sensory receptors, calming your nervous system. This kind of stimulation is crucial, especially if you're battling chronic stress or anxiety. It's like whispering a soothing lullaby to your nervous system, telling it to slow down, unwind, and switch from fight-or-flight mode to a state of rest and digest. Activating this state reduces stress, enhances digestion, and lowers heart rate, fostering overall well-being.

Types of Touch Therapy

Let's explore various touch therapies that can help activate your vagus nerve, each offering unique benefits:

- **Skin-on-Skin Contact**: Sometimes, the simple act of human touch, whether a hug from a loved one or even a handshake, can initiate comfort and safety signals through your vagus nerve. This contact releases oxytocin, often called the 'love hormone,' which reduces cortisol levels and boosts mood.
- **Therapeutic Massage**: More structured than casual touch, therapeutic massages involve manipulating the body's soft tissues with techniques like kneading, tapping, rocking, and stroking. These techniques ease muscle tension and significantly enhance vagal activity, improving the parasympathetic nervous system's ability to calm the body and mind.
- **Acupressure**: This technique involves applying pressure to specific points on the body, mirroring acupuncture except without the needles. These points are junctures of energy channels, which, when stimulated, can release muscle tension and improve blood flow, enhancing vagal tone.

- **Acupuncture**: Thin needles inserted into the body's meridian points strategically align with your nerve pathways, stimulating the vagus nerve and encouraging healing and pain relief.
- **Craniosacral Therapy**: This gentle, non-invasive form of bodywork addresses the bones of the head, spinal column, and sacrum. The goal is to release compression in these areas, soothing pain and stress, which, in turn, enhances the function of the cerebrospinal fluid and the vagus nerve.
- **Reflexology**: Reflexology applies pressure to specific reflex points, primarily on the feet, hands, and ears, which correspond to organs and systems throughout the body. This pressure promotes relaxation and stimulates the vagus nerve, improving overall health.

SELF-MASSAGE TECHNIQUES FOR VAGUS NERVE STIMULATION

Imagine finding a quiet moment in your bustling day, a moment just for you, where, with simple movements of your own hands, you can profoundly change your body's state of relaxation and well-being. Self-massage is a gateway to such transformations, harnessing your intrinsic ability to calm the vagus nerve and enhance your parasympathetic nervous system's response. It's not just about easing muscle tension—it's about calming your nervous system, improving digestion, and soothing your heart rate.

The vagus nerve meanders through various parts of your body, but certain areas are particularly rich in vagal pathways. Two key areas are your neck and feet. Massaging these areas can stimulate the vagus nerve directly, promoting a cascade of relaxation responses throughout your body. In the neck, where the vagus nerve surfaces behind the ear, gentle circular motions with slight pressure can be profoundly soothing. Similarly, massaging the soles of your feet, with their abundant nerve endings, feels incredibly relaxing and helps activate vagal responses through spinal pathways.

Engaging in regular self-massage offers numerous benefits. It's a powerful tool for managing anxiety, reducing stress, and improving sleep quality by regularly calming your nervous system. Over time, these moments of self-induced peace can lead to a consistently higher vagal tone. Furthermore, self-massage can improve blood circulation, remove toxins from the lymphatic system, and enhance skin and tissue health, providing a holistic practice beneficial for the mind and body.

While professional massages offer depth and therapeutic intensity, self-massage provides a practical, budget-friendly, and immediate alternative that can be applied anytime, anywhere. The main advantage of self-massage is its accessibility; it allows you to respond to your body's needs spontaneously, enabling you to maintain and enhance vagal tone regularly and independently.

Self-Massage Techniques

Building a personal toolkit of self-massage techniques can be likened to assembling essential tools that keep your home functioning smoothly. Each tool serves a unique purpose, addressing different needs and areas of tension in your body.

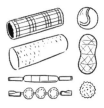 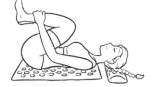

Here are some tools and techniques to consider:

- **Foam Rolling and Body Rolling**: These techniques utilize cylindrical rollers to apply pressure across large muscle groups, aiding muscle relaxation and fascia release. Rolling movements help stimulate blood flow and can be particularly soothing for tight legs or a stiff back. Vibrating options are now available.

- **Massage Balls and Self-Massage Tools**: Smaller than foam rollers, massage balls or tools like the Theracane allow for more localized pressure and are ideal for reaching deeper knots or specific points, such as the arches of your feet or the base of your neck.

- **TENS Units and Hand-Held Percussion Massagers**: These electronic devices offer a deeper level of stimulation through electrical pulses or rhythmic percussion, effectively mimicking the kneading hands of a massage therapist. They are beneficial for reducing deep muscle tension and improving local circulation.

- **Acupressure Mats and Pillows**: Lying on an acupressure mat or pillow can stimulate multiple points along your back or neck, offering a passive yet effective way to release tension and activate the vagus nerve through mild, steady pressure.

- **Cupping Devices**: Using glass or silicone cups to create suction on the skin is an ancient technique that promotes healing by drawing blood to the surface and easing muscle tension. This method can be particularly effective for areas that are difficult to address with hand massage alone.

While self-massage is generally safe, it's essential to approach it with awareness and care, especially if you have underlying health conditions. Always ensure that the pressure applied is comfortable and not causing pain. Avoid massaging areas where you have wounds, severe varicose veins, or recent fractures. Listen to your body's signals, and if you experience any discomfort or pain, adjust your technique or consult a professional.

SEXUAL HEALING: RELEASING THROUGH CLIMAX

In the vibrant tapestry of experiences that our bodies can offer, sexual activity is one of the most intense and profound. It's not just about pleasure; it's about connection, release, and a deep form of communication that occurs at the level of the nervous system. For many, this aspect of human experience remains mysterious, particularly in understanding how sexual climax interacts with our body's systems. The connection between orgasm and the stimulation of the vagus nerve offers fascinating insights into how sexual activity influences everything from our heart rate to our mood.

When you experience an orgasm, it's not just your heart that races and your breathing that quickens; your vagus nerve activates intensely, releasing neurotransmitters that profoundly impact your body. This release includes dopamine and oxytocin, which elevate your mood and create feelings of contentment and connection. It's a natural and powerful way to reduce stress and anxiety; these neurotransmitters help lower blood pressure and calm your body. Additionally, this chemical release provides natural pain relief and is beneficial for chronic pain conditions.

Sexual activity's impact on the vagus nerve also involves activating the parasympathetic nervous system—the part of your autonomic nervous system that helps you relax and recuperate. During sexual activity, particularly at climax, this system experiences significant stimulation, promoting calm and relaxation. This result holds whether engaging in sexual activities with a partner or through solo exploration. The physical and emotional intimacy involved, coupled with the fantasy or visualization that often accompanies sexual activity, enhances this effect, making the experience both pleasurable and therapeutically beneficial.

However, it's crucial to underscore the importance of safe and consensual touch in these interactions. Safe, consensual touch is essential not only for comfort and security but because it is the only context in which the body can fully relax and engage the parasympathetic responses that activate the vagus nerve effectively. For individuals who have experienced sexual trauma, reclaiming this aspect of vagal stimulation can be challenging. Mindful, consensual sexual practices can be a powerful part of healing, helping rewire associations of touch to create new pathways of safety and pleasure.

These stories highlight a critical yet often overlooked aspect of our health: the role of sexual health and fulfillment as a fundamental component of our overall well-being. As you explore the potential of sexual activity to enhance your vagal tone and promote health, remember to approach this exploration with sensitivity, respect boundaries, and emphasize safety and consent. Doing so opens a pathway to greater pleasure and a deeper, more profound sense of healing and connection.

THE POWER OF TOUCH: UNCONVENTIONAL OPPORTUNITIES

Every touch, whether a gentle brush against a leaf or the comforting pressure of a weighted blanket, can be a moment of healing as you navigate through your day. Recognizing the profound connection between our sense of touch and the nervous system's responses opens up a realm of accessible and powerful self-care possibilities, regardless of your relational or financial status. Often underestimated, the power of touch can transform ordinary interactions into opportunities for significant emotional and physical health benefits.

Imagine transforming every handshake into a moment of genuine human contact through the simple act of awareness. By altering your perspective slightly, what was once a perfunctory interaction becomes a comforting 'hand-hug.' This shift enlivens your daily interactions and stimulates your vagus nerve, promoting happiness and reducing stress. It's about finding joy and therapeutic value in the simple and sometimes mundane connections that fill your day.

For those who are single, elderly, or constrained by a tight budget, regular access to professional therapeutic touch like massages might not be feasible. The need for physical connection is a basic human right. Simple yet effective alternatives exist that can help bridge this gap. Engaging with animals offers a beautiful opportunity to enjoy the benefits of touch. Whether you arrange playdates with friends who have pets, spend time at local animal shelters, or visit petting zoos, petting animals can significantly boost your mood and vagal tone, thanks to the release of oxytocin, the 'cuddle hormone.'

For individuals experiencing isolation, community groups or events can provide opportunities for warm, platonic exchanges. Reconsider your opportunities to offer a hug—it is a powerful tool in your arsenal of touch. Extending a hug instead of a handshake deepens your connections and activates your parasympathetic nervous system, helping your body relax and rejuvenate. Additionally, using weighted blankets can mimic the pressure of a hug, offering comfort and alleviating anxiety from home.

Another delightful way to engage your sense of touch is through tactile adventures. Set aside time for a 15-minute walk where your sole focus is to explore different textures around you—feel the bark of trees, the texture of a cinderblock retaining wall or the weave of fabric while perusing items at the store. Each texture you encounter is not just a physical sensation but also a therapeutic interaction

that stimulates your vagus nerve, promoting calm and mindfulness.

TESTIMONIES OF TRANSFORMATION

The transformative power of touch therapies shines through
the experiences of those who have embraced them. These
stories illustrate the profound impact of nurturing touch on
the vagus nerve, showcasing its potential to recalibrate our
body's responses to stress, pain, and illness. Incorporating
touch therapies into your healing regimen isn't just about
alleviating symptoms—it's about reconnecting with your
body's innate ability to heal and find balance. As you explore
these modalities, remember that each gentle stroke or pressure point is a step towards a more harmonized state of
health, where your body and mind can flourish.

Bodywork and touch therapies offer profound healing
through physical touch and manipulation. Here are inspiring
stories of individuals who benefited from these practices.

Mark's Relaxation with Craniosacral Therapy: Mark, a
60-year-old retired veteran dealing with hypertension and
chronic migraines, was desperate for a solution that didn't
involve prescription drugs. A recommendation from the VA
led him to try craniosacral therapy. To his surprise, the gentle
manipulations were profoundly relaxing. Although he didn't
fully understand the mechanics, the relief he felt after one
session was undeniable, prompting him to schedule more
treatments. At his next VA appointment, his doctor noted a
significant reduction in his blood pressure and no new reports
of migraines. This therapy became a key component of

Mark's health regimen, significantly enhancing his overall quality of life and bringing him a profound sense of peace and rejuvenation.

Maria's Discovery of Joy with Tactile Stimulation: Maria, 53, struggled with feelings of loneliness and depression as a new empty-nester. Without the familiar demands of child-rearing and transporting to various activities, she felt a void in purpose and pleasure. She decided to fill some of her downtime by exploring local nurseries, enjoying the textures and smells of various plants. She found great joy in caressing the velvety soft "Lamb's Ear" plant, running her hands through ornamental grasses, and pinching the leaves of herbs to smell their fragrance. These trips became anchors of peace and happiness, evolving into a flourishing hobby caring for all the plants she brought home.

Adam's Grounding with Touch: Adam, 39, overwhelmed with grief over the loss of his young wife, became inspired by one of their son's fidget toys. He recalled a small bag of stones his wife collected from beaches during family vacations. Every morning, he selected a stone from the bag and put it in his pocket. Whenever emotions bubbled up at work, he would hold the stone, exploring its temperature and texture. This small action helped him stay present and feel connected to his departed wife through the shared experience of the memento. Years later, he continues with this routine as it brings him great joy to honor his wife in his self-care routine.

Reflecting on my own journey, particularly after the traumatic loss of my home in the CZU wildfire, I found solace and healing in the simple act of self-massage. Familiarity breeds comfort. At a time when all of that was stripped away, the only sense of comfort and familiarity I could find was in coming home to myself. Rebuilding my self-care toolkit became a priority to manage stress, modulate my nervous system, and take a mental break from the relentless demands of insurance claims, resource centers, and the intense work of rebuilding life from the ground up. Each evening, as I lay down, exploring which part of my body needed attention, I engaged in a healing dialogue with myself, using tools like massage balls and foam rollers to ease the day's tensions. This routine not only helped me relax; it became an important ritual to reclaim my sense of comfort and control during a time of immense upheaval and stress.

These stories highlight how, with creativity and openness, everyday interactions and objects can become powerful tools for wellness. Incorporating playful and therapeutic touch into your routine enhances physical and emotional health and deepens your connection with the world around you. This chapter reminds us that opportunities to heal and connect through touch are all around us—we only need to reach out and embrace them.

CHAPTER 17
COLD AND THERMAL EXPOSURE

THE POWER OF COLD EXPOSURE: SHOCKING THE SYSTEM

S tepping into a stream of chilly water, you feel an initial shock like electricity through your body, followed by a surprising calm. Cold exposure isn't just a test of willpower; it's a scientifically backed practice that can rejuvenate your nervous system, enhance your mood, and boost your immune response. This section explores the stimulating world of cold exposure, a therapy that offers profound benefits for those brave enough to embrace its chill.

When you subject your body to cold, it does more than just make you shiver. This experience activates the vagus nerve, which plays a crucial role in initiating the 'diving reflex,' an evolutionary adaptation that conserves oxygen and prioritizes blood flow to essential organs when submerged in cold water. This reflex slows your heart rate while increasing HRV, diverts blood to major organs, and conserves oxygen, leading to decreased stress levels, a stronger immune response, and an improved mood.

Cold exposure stimulates the release of norepinephrine, a natural chemical in the brain that acts as both a neurotransmitter and a hormone. Norepinephrine is essential in mobilizing the brain and body for action. In controlled cold exposure, it fosters calm and resilience. The body increases norepinephrine production by up to fivefold, reducing inflammation and pain while enhancing mood and vigilance, providing a natural boost of energy and alertness.

Additionally, cold exposure activates brown adipose tissue (BAT), or brown fat, which burns energy to generate heat, enhancing metabolic rate and improving insulin sensitivity. This thermogenic process releases beneficial hormones and cytokines that enhance overall metabolic health. Exposure to cold also triggers the production of cold shock proteins, such as RNA-binding motif protein 3 (RBM3), which plays a role in neuroprotection and synapse regeneration, enhancing cognitive function and protecting against neurodegenerative diseases.

Regular cold exposure can also strengthen the immune system by increasing the production of white blood cells and natural killer cells. These cells play a crucial role in defending the body against infections and diseases. Enhanced immune function results in fewer illnesses and quicker recovery times.

The biological responses to cold are multifaceted and interconnected. Cold exposure increases norepinephrine production, activates brown adipose tissue, triggers cold shock proteins, and stimulates the vagus nerve. These processes collectively reduce inflammation, enhance mood, improve metabolic health, boost immune function, and contribute to overall physical and mental well-being. Incorporating cold exposure into your routine can revitalize your nervous system, enhance mental clarity, and strengthen your body's resilience to stress and illness. Notably, the Wim Hof Method, which combines cold exposure with specific breathing techniques and meditation, exemplifies how harnessing cold can lead to remarkable improvements in health and resilience.

TYPES OF COLD EXPOSURE

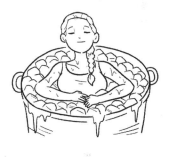

The methods of introducing your body to cold vary, each with unique intensity and approach. Cold showers are perhaps the most accessible form of cold therapy. Starting your morning with a cold shower can invigo-rate your vagus nerve and kickstart your day with heightened alertness and reduced anxiety. Ice baths or cold plunges, often embraced by athletes, help drastically reduce muscle soreness and improve recovery times. The pricing of cold plunge tanks have come down drastically in recent years, making them an effective home remedy.

Cryotherapy, another modern method, involves exposing the body to icy cold air for several minutes, helping relieve pain, inflammation, and even aid in weight loss. For a gentler introduction, you might try cold face immersion—splashing your face with cold water to stimulate the vagus nerve gently. Cold water swimming offers the combined benefits of physical activity and cold exposure, providing mental clarity from being in nature.

RESEARCH FINDINGS

Research supports the benefits of cold exposure, particularly its ability to activate the vagus nerve, which regulates the body's stress response. A study published in the Journal of Clinical Investigation showed that regular cold exposure significantly increased parasympathetic activity, the part of the nervous system responsible for rest and digestion. Participants reported decreased stress levels, improved mood, and heightened alertness. This research underscores the physiological transformations that come from routine cold exposure, highlighting an increase in the adaptive capacity of the nervous system.

Research from the University of Copenhagen reveals that routine cold immersion increases the production of white blood cells and antioxidants, crucial markers of an improved immune response. Participants in these studies also reported fewer colds and flu-like symptoms, adding to the growing body of evidence that cold exposure can boost immune function. This enhanced immune response is likely due to the body's adaptive mechanisms to the stress of cold, which helps fortify its defenses against pathogens.

Cold exposure is also shown to activate brown adipose tissue (BAT), or brown fat, which burns calories to generate heat and improves metabolic health. This activation can lead to better insulin sensitivity and a more efficient metabolic rate.

Additionally, exposure to cold triggers the production of cold shock proteins like RNA-binding motif protein 3 (RBM3), which plays a role in neuroprotection and synapse regeneration. This process enhances cognitive function and offers protection against neurodegenerative diseases.

The release of norepinephrine during cold exposure is another significant benefit. Norepinephrine acts as both a neurotransmitter and a hormone, essential for brain and body mobilization. Controlled cold exposure can increase norepinephrine levels up to fivefold, leading to reduced inflammation, decreased pain, and improved mood and vigilance. This natural boost of energy and alertness contributes to overall mental health and resilience.

Stepping out of our temperature comfort zones can lead to new health possibilities. Cold exposure, underpinned by science and real-world successes, is vital to unlocking a healthier, more vibrant version of ourselves. As we explore and understand these effects, we open new pathways for wellness that are both ancient in their origins and innovative in their application.

Our bodies thrive under healthy stress, and cold exposure is a powerful example of this. By embracing the chill, we harness our natural capacity for adaptation and growth, leading to profound health benefits and enhanced resilience.

SAFETY CONSIDERATIONS

While the benefits of cold exposure are compelling, it's crucial to approach this practice with caution and respect for your body's limits. Gradual adaptation techniques are essential. Start with brief, controlled exposure, such as a 30-second cold shower, gradually increasing the duration as your body adapts. Combining these practices with deep breathing is vital to help manage the initial shock and monitor your body's response.

Always consult a healthcare provider if you have underlying health conditions, such as cardiovascular issues, and never force yourself to endure extreme cold without proper progression. Ensure a warm environment is accessible when exiting the experience for a gradual and comfortable return to normal body temperature. Engage in cold exposure practices several times a week, allowing your body to build tolerance and resilience over time.

TESTIMONIES OF TRANSFORMATION

Cold and thermal exposure therapies can enhance resilience and reduce stress. The following stories highlight the benefits of these practices.

David's Playful Approach to Healing: David, 35, a nurse struggling with chronic fatigue, poor concentration, and brain fog, was anxious for a solution. His Naturopathic Doctor recommended cold showers as part of his health protocol. Initially skeptical, he started with 30 seconds of cold water at the end of his shower, gradually increasing the duration. He began to enjoy the refreshing and vigorous rush of the cold showers, feeling more alert and focused throughout the day. Amazed, he started seeing other opportunities for cold therapy, making a game out of staying in the walk-in fridge for 3-5 minutes every time he shopped at Costco. His playful approach to cold therapy reshaped his mindset around self-care as being fun instead of a chore.

Jamal's Relief with Cold Plunging Jamal, a 42-year-old construction worker dealing with rheumatoid arthritis, began using cold packs on his inflamed joints. Encouraged by the relief they provided, he began jumping in the local lake after work during the winter. He even got his buddies to partake in the challenge as they were all fascinated by both his physical improvement and happier attitude. As the warmer weather of summer approached, Jamal decided to invest in a home cold plunge tank to continue managing inflammation and pain on his terms. This practice helped Jamal manage his symptoms and maintain his physical activity levels.

These personal stories and scientific data blend to form a rich tapestry of evidence and inspiration in the evolving narrative of health and wellness. Especially with something as physically intense and beneficial as cold exposure, these stories illustrate the potential health benefits and provide a roadmap for those curious to try this method themselves. Embrace these practices and discover the incredible potential of engaging with your body's natural healing processes.

CHAPTER 18
BIOFEEDBACK AND TECHNOLOGY

S tep into a realm where you can feel, understand, and harness every subtle change in your heartbeat, every shift in your breathing, and every nuance of your body's responses for healing. Biofeedback technology offers a mirror reflecting the physiological processes typically hidden from conscious awareness. This chapter will guide you through the empowering world of biofeedback, showcasing how this technology can become a pivotal ally in your quest to optimize your vagus nerve health, enhance your well-being, and transform your approach to personal health management.

BIOFEEDBACK: HARNESSING TECHNOLOGY FOR VAGAL TONE

In Chapter 4, we explored biofeedback as a powerful diagnostic tool in clinical settings, revealing insights into the body's internal communications and pinpointing areas needing therapeutic attention. However, you can also access biofeedback from the comfort of your home and integrate it into your daily wellness routine.

Home biofeedback devices offer real-time data about your body's stress levels, heart rate variability (HRV), and muscle tension, allowing you to manage your health actively. These devices capture physiological data and provide simple, understandable metrics, educating you about your body's responses and empowering you to take proactive steps to manage stress, anxiety, and other conditions affecting your vagal tone.

Advancements in technology have made biofeedback devices more accessible and user-friendly for home use. Whether wearables monitoring HRV or compact devices tracking breathing patterns, these tools seamlessly integrate into daily life, enabling a routine of self-care informed by real-time, personalized biological feedback.

The benefits of incorporating biofeedback into your life are substantial. Biofeedback sheds light on normally invisible processes in your body, providing a unique training ground for developing greater control over your physiological responses. Through biofeedback, you can learn to alter your breathing patterns to directly affect your HRV. Over time, this practice improves emotional regulation, enhances relaxation, and reduces symptoms of stress and anxiety.

Beyond HRV, biofeedback can help manage chronic pain by teaching you to recognize and control the physical responses associated with pain. This tool can be particularly beneficial for conditions like migraines, fibromyalgia, and other pain disorders. By monitoring muscle tension, you can identify stress-related patterns and implement relaxation techniques to alleviate discomfort.

Biofeedback also plays a significant role in improving sleep quality. By tracking variables such as breathing patterns, heart rate, and skin temperature, you can identify factors disrupting your sleep and apply biofeedback techniques to create a more conducive environment for restful sleep.

Additionally, biofeedback can help manage high blood pressure. By understanding how your body responds to stress, you can practice relaxation techniques that promote vasodilation and lower blood pressure. These techniques improve cardiovascular health and reduce the risk of stroke and heart disease.

For individuals with anxiety disorders, biofeedback provides a way to monitor and control physiological reactions to anxiety triggers. The heightened awareness and control can lead to a significant reduction in panic attacks and generalized anxiety symptoms.

As your awareness of your body's signals improves, so does your ability to manage potential stressors preemptively, leading to a more balanced and health-oriented approach to daily challenges. Biofeedback fosters a deeper connection between mind and body, encouraging mindfulness and a proactive approach to health. Whether dealing with physical ailments or psychological stress, biofeedback equips you with the tools to improve your well-being and quality of life.

Biofeedback's versatility extends into therapeutic settings, particularly for conditions like hypertension, where maintaining a balanced vagal tone is crucial. For individuals dealing with high blood pressure, regular biofeedback sessions focusing on relaxation and stress management can lead to significant improvements. The data collected during these sessions can help you and your healthcare provider develop more effective, personalized management plans, adjusting treatments based on your body's responses.

By transforming abstract physiological data into understandable, actionable information, biofeedback bridges the scientific understanding of bodily functions with practical, everyday health practices. It invites you to a closer relationship with yourself, fostering a deeper engagement with your body's signals. This connection creates an environment where you actively pursue healing and well-being in the comfort of your own space.

Embarking on biofeedback at home begins with selecting the right tool. When choosing a biofeedback device, consider what physiological parameters you want to monitor—heart rate, muscle tension, or brain waves. Look for devices that track these metrics and provide clear, actionable insights you can use to improve your health.

Once you have your device, integrating it into your daily routine is critical. Start with short, consistent sessions focusing on reading and interpreting the feedback. Gradually, as you become more attuned to understanding and controlling your physiological responses, extend these sessions and experiment with different techniques to enhance your vagal tone, such as focused breathing or mindfulness meditation.

TESTIMONIES OF TRANSFORMATION

Biofeedback and technology-based therapies offer innovative ways to monitor and improve health. These stories illustrate how individuals have benefited from these advancements, transforming their health and well-being through active engagement with cutting-edge technology.

Alex's Control with HRV Monitoring: Alex, a 42-year-old IT professional with generalized anxiety disorder, started using an HRV monitor to track his heart rate variability. By observing his stress levels and incorporating relaxation techniques, Alex gained better control over his anxiety. The HRV monitor provided real-time feedback, empowering him to make informed decisions about his health and well-being. This technology transformed Alex's approach to managing anxiety, leading to a more balanced and confident life.

Jordon's Relief with TENS Unit: Jordon, a 36-year-old former athlete, suffered a severe knee injury that led to chronic pain and depression. He found relief through neuromodulation with transcutaneous nerve stimulation (TENS), using the device on the muscles supporting his knee and to stimulate the vagus nerve. The mild electrical impulses helped him manage pain perception and speed recovery time. As hope and healing took hold, his depressive symptoms naturally lifted.

Priya's Sleep Improvement with Sleep Tracker and VNS Device: Priya, a 46-year-old creative writer dealing with panic attacks and insomnia, sought a solution through biofeedback technology. She started using a sleep tracker and a personal

VNS device to understand and improve her sleep patterns. The data from the sleep tracker revealed her baseline sleep issues, while the VNS device helped promote relaxation. This combination significantly reduced Priya's insomnia and panic attacks, giving her greater control over her sleep quality and mental health.

These personal stories illustrate the potential health benefits of cold exposure and provide a roadmap for those curious to try this method themselves. Embrace these practices and discover the incredible potential of engaging with your body's natural healing processes.

CHAPTER 19

EMOTIONAL AND SOCIAL HEALING

THE ROLE OF LAUGHTER AND SOCIAL INTERACTION

Picture this: you're gathered with friends, sharing stories and laughs that echo through the room, uplifting everyone's spirits. It's more than just fun; it's therapeutic. In these moments, your body creates a powerful wave of responses that enhance your mood and bolster your health. Understanding the impact of laughter and social interactions on your vagus nerve provides profound insights into the deep interconnection between our emotions and physiological health.

Laughter as a Catalyst for Healing

Laughter, often called the best medicine, has tangible benefits beyond fleeting joy. When you laugh, you activate a cascade of positive reactions in your body. It begins with an increase in the intake of oxygen-rich air, stimulating your heart, lungs, and muscles. Laughter initiates a significant activation of the vagus nerve, which triggers the release of endorphins, your body's natural feel-good chemicals.

These endorphins lead to a temporary decrease in the perception of pain and increased feelings of well-being. Additionally, laughter can reduce stress hormones such as cortisol and adrenaline, calming your nervous system. This response promotes relaxation and healing, which is why you might experience relief, reduced anxiety, or a more positive outlook after a good laugh.

The Power of Social Connections

Positive social interactions play a crucial role in enhancing vagal tone, a key factor in managing stress and promoting recovery from health issues. Engaging with others, feeling understood, and sharing experiences help activate the vagus nerve, fostering a sense of safety and belonging that leads to calming and therapeutic effects.

Research consistently highlights the importance of social connections for both mental and physical health. For example, studies on *Blue Zones*—areas where people live significantly longer and healthier lives—show that strong social ties are a common factor among these communities. Individuals with deep, meaningful connections have lower rates of chronic illnesses and higher overall well-being.

A study published in *Psychosomatic Medicine* found that individuals with robust social support systems had significantly higher heart rate variability (HRV) compared to those with weaker social ties. Higher HRV is associated with better stress resilience and overall cardiovascular health, suggesting that nurturing quality connections can enhance your body's ability to manage stress.

Additionally, social connections are vital for mental health. Research published in *The American Journal of Psychiatry* indicates that people with strong social networks are less likely to experience loneliness and depression. Engaging in meaningful social activities can provide emotional support and reduce the risk of mental health issues, contributing to a more balanced emotional state.

Furthermore, incorporating social activities and laughter into your daily routine can have substantial long-term health benefits. Studies have shown that individuals who maintain strong social bonds and engage in regular laughter experience lower levels of inflammation, better immune responses, and a reduced risk of heart disease. Laughter, often triggered by social interactions, activates the parasympathetic nervous system, which can lower blood pressure and reduce stress hormones.

It's important to note that cultivating these connections doesn't require constant socialization. Instead, focus on quality interactions that bring joy and comfort. By embracing the power of social connections and integrating laughter and shared experiences into your life, you're not only enhancing your mood but also actively building a foundation for better health and emotional resilience. This holistic approach empowers you to make daily choices that foster both physical and emotional well-being.

Integrating Laughter and Social Engagement into Your Life

To harness the benefits of laughter and social interactions, engage in activities that incorporate both. Laughter yoga, which combines laughter exercises with yogic breathing, is an excellent example. It helps stimulate the vagus nerve through laughter and enhances lung capacity and oxygen intake.

Regular meet-ups with friends are essential for emotional and physical health. Support groups and community activities foster a sense of belonging and shared experience. Creating opportunities for laughter in these gatherings elevates the benefits for all. Arranging game nights, attending comedy clubs, taking improv classes with friends, or starting a group dedicated to writing and telling jokes are fun ways to infuse laughter into your life. Starting a book club focused on humorous books, hosting a costumed pet parade, or organizing themed costume events with funny awards like "Best Laugh" or "Most Elaborate Costume" can bring silliness into your life and the lives of others. Try "The Smallest Smile" game with friends for a fun and playful activity. Take turns competing to make the smallest possible smile using your facial muscles. This game taps into visualization and mindfulness exercises, helping you experience a smile more fully. It activates hormonal responses, providing the benefits of a full smile and often triggering bouts of actual laughter.

TESTIMONIES OF TRANSFORMATION

Emotional and social healing practices can significantly improve mental health and well-being. Here are stories of individuals who found healing through these methods.

Mia's Relief with Laughter Yoga

Mia, a 38-year-old writer struggling with chronic migraines, found profound relief through laughter yoga. The combination of laughter exercises and yogic breathing reduced the frequency and severity of her migraines and also provided a sense of community support. The social aspect further alleviated her stress, making her migraines more manageable and enhancing her overall well-being.

Minh's Improvement with Social Connections

Minh, a 31-year-old factory worker facing chronic pain and depression, discovered the healing power of social connections. By attending community events and social gatherings, he found solace and support in the shared experiences of others. These interactions significantly lifted his mood and eased his pain, transforming his outlook on life and bringing a sense of purpose and belonging.

These stories underscore the profound impact of laughter and social interactions on mental and physical health. Integrating these practices into your life can lead to significant improvements in well-being, resilience, and overall happiness. Embrace the power of laughter and connection to transform your health and enrich your life.

PART V: FUTURE DIRECTIONS

ESTABLISHING YOUR PRACTICE AND EXPLORING INNOVATIONS

CHAPTER 20

YOUR VNS ROUTINE
ESTABLISHING A LIFELONG PRACTICE

BUILDING YOUR VNS MORNING ROUTINE

S tarting each day with a calming ritual can set a tone of balance and resilience for the hours ahead. These practices stimulate the vagus nerve, a key player in regulating your body's relaxation responses, and help set your stress response to a baseline of calm. Think of it as tuning an instrument before a performance; this ensures that your physiological responses harmonize with your environment, enhancing your mood, digestion, and overall well-being throughout the day.

Simple Morning Exercises

To integrate vagus nerve stimulation into your morning, consider these five routines. Each one takes 10 to 20 minutes and combines techniques previously discussed in the book. Designed for flexibility, you can adapt them based on your morning schedule and specific needs.

Five-Minute Breathing and Gratitude Session (10 minutes total)

- Spend the first five minutes practicing diaphragmatic breathing, which directly stimulates the vagus nerve by increasing heart rate variability.
- Follow with five minutes of gratitude journaling or mental listing, which shifts your nervous system towards a positive emotional state, further calming the vagus nerve.

Gentle Yoga Flow with Meditative Focus (20 minutes)

- Engage in a 15-minute gentle yoga sequence, focusing on poses that open the chest and stimulate the neck area, where the vagus nerve is accessible.
- Conclude with a five-minute meditation, concentrating on the sensation of movement and breath, which enhances the calming effect on the vagus nerve.

Progressive Muscle Relaxation and Visualization (15 minutes)

- To reduce physical tension and stress, begin with ten minutes of progressive muscle relaxation, starting from your feet and moving up. Spend the last five minutes visualizing a serene place. This process can help your brain trigger incredible relaxation responses.

Humming and Stretching Routine (10 minutes)

- Spend five minutes humming your favorite tune, which vibrates the vocal cords and stimulates the vagus nerve.
- Follow with five minutes of dynamic stretching, focusing on neck rolls and shoulder shrugs that activate the muscle areas connected to vagal pathways.

Cold Shower and Affirmations (10 minutes)

- Start with a three-minute cold shower, which shocks the vagus nerve into reducing inflammation and boosting mood-enhancing neurotransmitters.
- Dry off and spend the next seven minutes reciting positive affirmations that set a purposeful tone for the day.

By incorporating these routines into your morning, you awaken your body holistically and healthfully and empower yourself to handle the day's stresses with grace and ease. Each activity is a stepping stone to a more resilient you, one morning at a time.

VNS FOR THE WORKPLACE: STRESS MANAGEMENT ON THE GO

Creating a workspace that feels like a refuge can significantly impact managing stress and maintaining your mental health throughout the workday. Consider the sensory environment of your workspace. Introducing sound-blocking headphones can transform your immediate area into a sanctuary of calm, shielding you from the chaotic symphony of office noises. Headphones are fabulous for creating silence but also for listening to binaural beats, which engage your vagus nerve in subtle yet profound ways, facilitating deep concentration and relaxation.

Organizing your desk with personal comfort items like plants, which bring a bit of nature's tranquility indoors, or photos that remind you of joyful moments. These items can subtly enhance your mood and reduce stress triggers. Each element in your workspace should serve a purpose: to inspire, calm, or energize you. The physical arrangement should allow for minimal clutter, promoting an environment where you can breathe and think clearly. Calm, clean surroundings support vagal health and make it easier to engage in stress-reducing practices without feeling overwhelmed.

Quick and discreet techniques to manage stress and stimulate your vagus nerve are invaluable tools during a busy workday. Simple breathing exercises, like the 4-7-8 technique, can be done right at your desk. This practice involves breathing in deeply for four seconds, holding the breath for seven seconds, and exhaling slowly for eight seconds. This method helps regulate the nervous system and can be particularly effective before or after stressful meetings or during a midday break. Mindfulness exercises, such as focusing on the sensations of your breath or briefly engaging in a guided meditation via a smartphone app, can also serve as a quick reset for your nervous system, fostering calm and focus amidst workplace challenges.

Moreover, developing stress-reducing habits that stack with your regular routines can significantly enhance your ability to maintain a high vagal tone throughout the day. For instance, make it a habit to stand up and stretch every 30 minutes, alleviating physical strain and re-engaging your nervous system. Pair this with a hydration habit—take a few sips of water each time you stand. Linking these actions together strengthens the routine and ensures you stay hydrated, further supporting overall health and cognitive function.

Another effective habit is incorporating humming or soft singing into regular breaks, leveraging the vagus nerve's accessibility via vocal cord vibration to calm your mind and body. If your environment allows, doing this while walking to the restroom or printer can multiply the benefits, as gentle physical movement stimulates the vagus nerve. For those who wear biofeedback devices, use the data as a prompt to engage in a quick visualization or breathing exercise whenever your stress markers rise. This immediate response helps regulate your stress levels in real-time, preventing them from escalating and disrupting your day.

Integrating these practices into your daily work routine establishes a cycle of continuous vagal stimulation and stress management, enhancing your productivity and supporting your overall health and well-being. This proactive approach allows you to handle workplace challenges with resilience and calm, transforming your professional environment into a space where you can thrive.

BUILDING YOUR VNS EVENING ROUTINE

In the quiet moments of the evening, as the world begins to slow, there is a precious opportunity to create a sanctuary of calm within your life. Establishing an evening routine dedicated to winding down can significantly influence your body's ability to transition smoothly into restorative sleep. Preparing the mind and body to rest and rejuvenate takes thoughtful planning. Engaging in practices that gently stimulate your vagus nerve sets the stage for deep relaxation, enhancing sleep quality and supporting overall health by regulating circadian rhythms and hormonal balance. Working toward waking up naturally without an alarm clock can further support your nervous system and promote a more balanced and peaceful start to your day.

Creating a relaxing environment is crucial. Dimming the lights, lighting calming scented candles, and playing soothing music signal to your nervous system that the day's demands are ending. This shift from daylight alertness to evening tranquility helps craft an atmosphere where stress dissolves and calm prevails, establishing a rhythm your body will recognize and respond to, night after night.

Simple Evening Exercises

To help you embrace this nightly calm, here are five structured routines, each designed to take 10 to 20 minutes, allowing you to end your day with intentional tranquility. These routines blend various techniques to engage the vagus nerve, promoting relaxation and preparing you for sleep.

Breathing and Reflective Reading (20 minutes)

- Spend the first 10 minutes engaged in slow, deep breathing exercises. Focus on inhaling deeply through your nose, holding for a few seconds, and exhaling slowly through your mouth. This type of breathing activates the vagus nerve, encouraging a state of calm throughout your body.
- For the next 10 minutes, read from a book that uplifts or relaxes you. Choose material that brings joy or peace, avoiding stimulating or distressing content before bed.

Gentle Yoga and Herbal Tea (20 minutes)

- Perform a 15-minute sequence of gentle yoga. Focus on poses that release tension in the neck, shoulders, and back, where stress accumulates. Poses like 'Child's Pose' and 'Legs-Up-The-Wall' can be particularly beneficial for activating the vagus nerve.
- Conclude your session with a warm herbal tea, such as chamomile or lavender. These teas aid in relaxation and digestion, complementing the vagal stimulation from yoga.

Guided Visualization and Aromatherapy (15 minutes)

- Engage in a 10-minute guided visualization exercise. Use an app or audio track that guides you to imagine a serene location, focusing on the sensory details of this peaceful place.

- Pair this practice with aromatherapy. Use essential oils such as lavender or sandalwood in a diffuser to enhance the calming effects of your visualization practice.

Journaling and Progressive Muscle Relaxation (15 minutes)

- Spend 5 minutes writing in a gratitude journal, reflecting on the positive aspects of your day. This practice shifts your focus away from stress and fosters a positive mindset.
- Follow with 10 minutes of progressive muscle relaxation. Tense and then relax each muscle group, starting from your toes and moving up to your head, which can significantly reduce physical tension and stimulate the vagus nerve.

Meditation and Deep Breathing (10 minutes)

- Engage in a 5-minute meditation, focusing on clearing your mind and deepening your breath. A simple mindfulness practice where you observe your thoughts without attachment is perfect.
- Follow with 5 minutes of deep breathing exercises, emphasizing exhalation to activate the vagus nerve and enhance relaxation.

These evening routines are not just rituals; they are tools that actively engage your vagus nerve, promoting physiological changes that enhance sleep quality. By regulating your circadian rhythm and supporting hormonal balance, these practices help align your body's natural sleep readiness with nighttime, resulting in deeper, more restorative sleep, crucial for recovery and health.

To maximize the benefits of your evening routine, declare your bedroom a technology-free zone. This means no smartphones, tablets, or laptops. The blue light emitted by screens can interfere with melatonin production, the hormone responsible for regulating sleep. By eliminating these sources of blue light, you protect your circadian rhythm, making it easier for your body to wind down naturally. In this space, where calm reigns and technology fades into the background, your body finds the peace it needs to rejuvenate fully, guided by the gentle hand of your vagus nerve.

STRESS-BUSTING ROUTINES: QUICK FIXES FOR HIGH-PRESSURE MOMENTS

Finding peace can feel nearly impossible during a bustling day or a sudden surge of stress. Yet, precisely within these moments, your body needs a break. A short routine, compact yet potent, can significantly shift your nervous system away from the edge of overwhelm and towards a state of tranquility. Here, I'll guide you through a simple 10-minute routine designed to quickly recalibrate your system, emphasizing the vagus nerve's role in restoring balance. This routine is your quick escape hatch from stress, a way to reset and refresh no matter where you are or what's happening around you.

Quick Breathing Exercises: The Power of the 4-7-8 Technique (2 minutes)

Start with a breathing technique that's deceptively simple but profoundly effective. The 4-7-8 breathing method, a rhythmic pattern that promotes relaxation, can be done anywhere, anytime. Here's how it works: comfortably inhale through your nose for a count of four, allowing your abdomen, not just your chest, to rise as you fill your lungs. Hold this breath for seven seconds—a pause that allows oxygen to saturate your bloodstream. Then, exhale slowly through your mouth for eight seconds, releasing more carbon dioxide from your lungs than a regular breath. This controlled breathing helps regulate the heart rate and directly stimulates the vagus nerve, enhancing its ability to usher in calm. Repeat this cycle three times to initiate your body's relaxation response.

Progressive Muscle Relaxation: Releasing Tension from Head to Toe (2 minutes)

Next, transition into progressive muscle relaxation (PMR), a practice that reduces stress and physical tension by sequentially tensing and relaxing different muscle groups. This technique heightens your awareness of physical sensations and encourages deep relaxation. Begin by focusing on the muscles in your feet. Tense them as much as you can for five seconds, then release all that pent-up energy, noticing the following warmth and lightness. Gradually move up your body—calves, thighs, abdomen, chest, arms, and face. Each muscle group follows the same tense-and-release pattern. PMR not only relaxes your muscles but also sends signals to your brain to calm down, further activating the vagus nerve and deepening your state of relaxation.

Quick Physical Movement: Shoulder Rolls and Neck Stretches (2 minutes)

Incorporate some gentle physical movements to release any remaining stiffness or stress. Begin with shoulder rolls, a simple yet effective way to relieve tension in your shoulders and neck—areas where stress commonly accumulates. Roll your shoulders slowly in a circular motion, five times forward, then five times backward. Follow this with neck stretches. Tilt your head to the left, holding the stretch for five seconds, feeling the stretch along the right side of your neck, then switch to the right. Repeat the movement, tilting your head forward and backward. If comfortable, add a gentle hum throughout these movements, a sound that vibrates in your throat and stimulates the vagus nerve, enhancing the calming effect of the stretches.

Mindfulness Moments: Grounding in the Present (2 minutes)

Mindfulness brings you back to the present moment, a powerful practice to diffuse stress. Spend two minutes on a simple grounding exercise that engages your senses, which can be particularly helpful if anxiety has made you feel detached or spaced out. Look around and note five things you can see: the color of the sky, the texture of your desk, or the face of a loved friend or pet. Touch four objects around you, feeling their temperature, texture, and weight. Listen for three distinct sounds, perhaps the hum of traffic, birdsong, or the quiet breaths you take. Identify two things you can smell: your coffee, a pencil, or a hint of perfume. Finally, focus on one thing you can taste, like a sip of water or the lingering flavor of your last meal. This sensory check-in brings a profound sense of here and now, significantly reducing feelings of overwhelm.

Affirmations and Positive Self-Talk: Cultivating Inner Peace (2 minutes)

Conclude your routine with affirmations, a potent tool for transforming your mental state. Affirmations reinforce positive thinking and can reshape the often negative internal narrative during stress. With a deep, grounding breath, affirm to yourself, "I am calm and in control." Repeat this three times, allowing the words to sink in and resonate. Add other affirmations, such as "I am capable of handling this" or "I am safe and relaxed." These statements aren't just words; they're a powerful declaration of your ability to manage your feelings and assert control over your emotional state.

This practical 10-minute routine engages the vagus nerve and swiftly guides you from stress to serenity. Whether at home, work, or anywhere in between, these techniques are quick, discreet, and incredibly effective in restoring peace and balance. Remember, the more you practice, the more second-nature these techniques will become, providing an immediate method of reclaiming calm in stressful situations.

ADVANCED TECHNIQUES FOR VAGAL TONE ENHANCEMENT

While all the techniques previously mentioned are undeniably effective, incorporating dynamic physical activities into your routine can dramatically enhance these efforts. Integrating high-intensity interval training (HIIT) with mindfulness or breathing techniques challenges your body and centers your mind, creating a powerful dual effect that maximizes physiological and psychological resilience.

Engaging in HIIT, combined with intentional VNS techniques, extends benefits beyond physical fitness. Your heart rate spikes during HIIT, and incorporating focused breathing exercises during rest periods rapidly activates your parasympathetic response. This practice enhances your body's ability to shift between high intensity and relaxation, directly training your vagal flexibility—a key factor in stress resilience and emotional regulation.

To deepen the impact of such physical routines, consider engaging in practices that enhance your mindfulness and meditation skills. Participating in silent retreats or advanced meditation courses can significantly impact your vagal health, teaching you to maintain calm and mindfulness amidst daily stresses. These experiences often introduce advanced breathing techniques that allow you to reach altered states of consciousness, further enhancing your control over stress responses.

Each component of this combined practice supports the others synergistically. Mindfulness reduces baseline stress levels, enhancing the effectiveness of physical exercises on your vagal tone. Linking breath to movement in exercises like yoga or targeted stretching within your HIIT routine supports the natural pump action of your diaphragm, directly stimulating your vagus nerve and enhancing relaxation. A positive feedback loop amplifies and speeds up results.

Leverage wearable technology to fine-tune these exercises for optimal vagal tone enhancement. Devices like the Whoop Strap or Oura Ring provide real-time feedback on your heart rate variability (HRV), a direct marker of your vagal tone. Biofeedback devices like the Heart Math or Muse Headband give you live insights into your physiological responses, allowing you to adjust your practices for maximum benefit. Integrate electrostimulation devices such as Apollo Neuro or Nervana into your routine for deeper nerve stimulation. Advanced sleep trackers like the Dream Headband help analyze the effectiveness of these practices on sleep patterns, providing a holistic view of health enhancement.

TESTIMONIALS OF TRANSFORMATION

When I was diagnosed with Mold Illness affecting multiple organ systems, I knew I needed a comprehensive approach to recovery. Guided by my Naturopath, I implemented a plan that included dietary changes, vagus nerve stimulation activities, supplements, medications, and detox protocols. This journey taught me the importance of balancing self-care practices with daily life.

A pivotal moment came when I combined breathwork with yoga, unlocking a new level of nervous system regulation. This combination increased my lung capacity and brought me into a coherent state, helping me to modulate stress responses more effectively. As a result, all my systems began to function better, and my overall health improved significantly.

The key takeaway from my experience is that the nervous system is central to effective self-care. From a down-regulated state of nervous system arousal, self-care is vastly more efficient and beneficial. So now I combine VNS with regular self-care: I hum while showering, recite affirmations during evening stretches, sing while cooking, and practice therapeutic shaking while waiting for my morning tea. I love to listen to binaural beats while working and the Giyatri or Prana Apana Mantra while driving. These small, consistent, synergistic practices have profoundly impacted my well-being.

For those eager to enhance their self-care, I recommend exploring the first book in the Revive and Thrive series, "The Ultimate Self Care Handbook: 1000+ Hassle-Free Ideas to Escape Burnout, Reduce Stress, and Reclaim Your Life." This book offers numerous ideas to personalize and balance your self-care routine, providing valuable insights for integrating vagal tone exercises into your lifestyle.

Contrary to the common myth that self-care is time-consuming or expensive, my experience shows that integrating VNS stimulation into everyday activities requires only a shift in focus and desire, making it accessible to everyone without adding extra time or cost.

CHAPTER 21

STAYING STRONG
MAINTAINING VAGUS NERVE HEALTH

P icture your body as a finely tuned instrument, with the vagus nerve as a string that vibrates with the rhythms of your daily activities, emotions, and interactions. Keeping this string finely tuned ensures that the music of your life plays smoothly, reflecting a state of health and balance. But how do you know if this vital nerve is in harmony with your body's needs? This chapter delves into practical and insightful methods to monitor, adjust, and maintain the health of your vagus nerve, empowering you to take control of your well-being in a hands-on, informed manner.

Monitoring Your Progress: Tools and Techniques

In the journey of maintaining and enhancing your vagal tone, the ability to measure progress isn't just helpful—it's crucial. It's like having a roadmap while navigating a complex network of roads; without it, you might not realize you've veered off-path until you're miles away from your destination. Heart rate variability (HRV) monitors are among the most effective tools. HRV measures the time variation between heartbeats, which the vagus nerve directly influences. Higher variability indicates healthier vagus nerve function, implying better stress resilience and cardiovascular health.

Utilizing devices like HRV monitors can provide immediate feedback about your body's response to various situations and practices. Whether following a guided breathing exercise, engaging in a yoga session, or navigating stressful events, your HRV scores can offer insightful data on how well your vagus nerve functions. By observing these patterns over time, you can start pinpointing which activities bolster your vagal tone and which ones might be causing stress, allowing for more tailored and effective routines.

Journaling for Reflection and Growth

Alongside technological tools, maintaining a journal can be a profoundly effective strategy for enhancing your vagal health. It's not just about recording events; it's about reflecting on your emotional and physiological responses to different scenarios. Each entry helps you to connect the dots between your feelings, the state of your body, and your vagus nerve's health. For instance, noting how relaxed and calm you feel after a meditation session or the tension during a hectic day can help you understand your body's cues and vagus nerve reactions more clearly.

Journaling cultivates heightened self-awareness, enabling you to notice subtle shifts in your well-being that you might miss otherwise. It encourages a deeper engagement with your vagal health practices, turning each activity into an opportunity for learning and adaptation. By documenting your experiences, you're not just keeping a record but crafting a personalized guide to your health.

Setting and Reviewing Goals: How to Stay on Track

Setting realistic and achievable goals is fundamental in any health regimen, especially when it involves the complex interplay of the vagus nerve within your body's systems. Initially, define clear, concise goals based on understanding your body's needs—perhaps enhancing sleep quality, managing anxiety, or improving digestive health through increased vagal tone. These goals should be clear and measurable, where tools like HRV monitors come into play, providing tangible metrics to track your progress.

Periodic review of these goals is just as important as setting them. Life changes, and so does your body. Regular check-ins on your goals allow you to adjust them in response to your progress and current circumstances. Maybe you've achieved your initial goals and are ready for more advanced challenges, or perhaps you've encountered obstacles that require you to scale back and refocus. These reviews align your practices with your body's needs, fostering continuous improvement and adaptation.

Feedback Loops and Adjustments: Fine-Tuning Your Practices

The true essence of maintaining your vagus nerve health lies in the feedback loops you establish from monitoring tools and personal reflection. This ongoing loop—action, monitoring, reflection, and adjustment—makes your approach to vagal health dynamic and responsive. For instance, if your HRV data shows less variability and your journal reflects a period of increased stress, you might incorporate more mindfulness exercises into your routine.

These adjustments are not about striving for perfection but making minor, informed tweaks that progressively enhance your well-being. This iterative process ensures that your approach to maintaining vagal health evolves like your life and health conditions. It empowers you to make informed decisions that keep your body's harmony intact, allowing the music of your life to play on beautifully without missing a beat.

Overcoming Common Obstacles and Maintaining Motivation

When you embark on a path to enhance your vagus nerve health, it's like nurturing a garden. You plant seeds (initiate practices), water them (nurture with consistency), and some-times, despite your best efforts, you hit roadblocks—pests, unforeseen weather, or the soil just isn't right. It's natural in any growth process.

Creating a support system can significantly enhance your journey. Just as plants in a garden thrive with the support of stakes and trellises, friends, family, or online communities can bolster your efforts to improve your vagal tone with encouragement and accountability. Connecting with others who share similar health goals or challenges can provide moral support, practical tips, and shared experiences that can be incredibly motivating. Whether it's joining a yoga class, participating in an online forum, or simply having a friend to discuss your progress with, these connections can be a powerful catalyst for sustained effort and success.

Keeping your practice fresh is crucial for maintaining long-term engagement. Just as a gardener rotates crops to optimize soil health, introduce variety into your VNS practices to keep your routine engaging and effective. Try new types of meditation, explore different genres of calming music for sound therapy, or switch up your diet to include new anti-inflammatory recipes. The key is to prevent your routine from becoming stagnant, which can lead to boredom and decreased motivation. Regularly introducing new elements ensures that your engagement remains high and your approach continues evolving with your changing needs and interests.

Regular review and revision of your health plan are akin to a gardener periodically assessing the health of their plants and soil. This practice helps you determine what's working, what isn't, and what adjustments might be necessary to enhance the effectiveness of your vagus nerve health regimen. Celebrating milestones along the way is important—acknowledging your progress, no matter how small can be incredibly uplifting and motivating. Whether it's improved sleep quality, reduced anxiety, or feeling more at peace, each success is a testament to your efforts and a reason to continue.

Maintaining an ongoing relationship with healthcare professionals can provide expert guidance tailored to your needs. Regular check-ups and discussions about your vagus nerve health practices can help optimize your approach, ensuring you get the most out of your efforts. These professionals can offer insights into the latest research, suggest adjustments to your routine, and provide encouragement and support throughout your health maintenance journey. Like a gardener consulting with a horticulturist to ensure the best care for their plants, working with healthcare providers ensures you are nurturing your vagus nerve health with the best knowledge and tools available.

The Role of Community and Social Engagement in Vagal Health

In the tapestry of life, the threads of social connections are as vital as the physical body itself. Consider how laughter with friends or a heartfelt conversation can lighten your spirits; this isn't just an emotional lift but also a physical one, where your vagus nerve plays a quietly decisive role. Social engagement does more than enrich your life—it actively stimulates your vagus nerve, enhancing your emotional and physical well-being. This nerve, your body's peacekeeper, thrives on positive social interactions, which release neurotransmitters like oxytocin, known as the 'love hormone,' soothing your heart rate and reducing stress.

Finding your tribe, a community that resonates with your interests and supports your well-being can be transformative. It's not just about having company but about enriching your life with relationships that encourage you to maintain and enhance your vagal health practices. Engaging with a community interested in vagal health practices can provide encouragement, new insights, and a greater collective wisdom than you might achieve alone. Whether it's a yoga class, a meditation group, or an online forum discussing the latest wellness practices, each interaction can stimulate your vagus nerve in ways that solitary practices might not.

Volunteering and altruism also play significant roles in this holistic health approach. Acts of kindness and helping others can activate your vagus nerve, reducing your heart rate and blood pressure and ultimately lowering stress levels. Studies have shown that people who regularly volunteer have better mental health and live longer. Engaging in community service provides a sense of purpose and fulfillment that goes beyond the immediate benefits, creating ripples of positive impact both personally and socially.

Group activities are particularly potent for vagal activation. Organizing workshops or participating in group exercises focusing on breathing techniques, mindfulness, or other vagal stimulation methods can amplify your efforts. The collective energy of a group, the shared breathing space, and the synchronized activities contribute to a heightened vagal tone for you and all participants. These gatherings are opportunities to learn, share, and grow together, reinforcing the practices that support vagal health in a fun and engaging way.

For those looking to cultivate or join a community, start by exploring local wellness events, online forums, or social media groups focused on vagal nerve health practices. Be proactive by attending seminars, joining clubs, or even starting your own group if one doesn't exist. Share your story, listen to others, and build connections that enrich your life and health.

As you weave these practices into the fabric of your daily life, remember that each social interaction, community engagement, and act of kindness is a step towards a healthier, more vibrant you. Keep exploring, connecting, and letting your vagus nerve thrive in the rich soil of community and social interaction. This exploration highlights a simple yet profound truth: as social beings, our health significantly intertwines with our interactions and community engagement, which is crucial for maintaining vagus nerve health. As you move forward, carry with you the understanding that your well-being is not just a personal journey but a communal dance. With this chapter as your guide, step confidently into the next, where we will delve into advanced techniques for vagus nerve stimulation, building upon the foundation laid here. Let's continue to nurture our collective well-being, empowered by knowledge and strengthened by community.

CHAPTER 22

THE FUTURE IS NOW

TECHNOLOGICAL ADVANCES IN VAGAL STIMULATION

I n a world where technology increasingly touches every aspect of our lives, it's not surprising that these advancements have reached the medical community. Powerful devices now exist to provide gentle electric impulses directly to the vagus nerve. These devices offer innovative solutions for alleviating anxiety, depression, seizures, digestive troubles, chronic pain, and inflammation. Supported by growing research and clinical trials to support their efficacy, these miracle devices are quickly becoming popularized.

ELECTRONIC VAGUS NERVE STIMULATORS: TYPES AND USES

Vagus nerve stimulation (VNS) technology has significantly matured, offering stable and effective treatment options. VNS devices can be broadly categorized into implantable and non-invasive options, each with specific applications and benefits.

Surgeons place implantable devices, such as the VNS Therapy® System, under the skin and connect them to the vagus nerve in the neck. These devices deliver continuous, controlled electrical pulses, making them highly effective for severe, chronic conditions like epilepsy and treatment-resistant depression. FDA-approved, these systems have demonstrated significant reductions in seizure frequency and improvements in depressive symptoms.

Non-invasive devices, such as the gammaCore®, target the cervical branch of the vagus nerve through the skin without requiring surgery. These user-friendly devices allow patients to manage their treatment at home and are particularly beneficial for conditions like migraines and chronic pain. The gammaCore® has received FDA approval for treating cluster headaches and migraines, supported by studies showing its effectiveness in reducing headache frequency and severity.

Choosing a suitable VNS device involves considering the severity and type of condition, lifestyle impacts, and comfort with medical procedures. Implantable devices provide consistent, long-term stimulation, ideal for persistent conditions, but they come with surgical risks and maintenance needs. Non-invasive devices offer flexibility and ease of use and are suitable for intermittent treatment but may require more frequent application. Regulatory approvals ensure these devices meet stringent safety and efficacy standards, giving confidence to patients and healthcare providers.

Vagus nerve stimulators represent the confluence of technology and medicine, offering innovative solutions for managing various health conditions. Understanding the types of VNS devices, their benefits, and their regulatory status allows patients and healthcare providers to make informed decisions aligned with individual health needs. These technological advances reflect a movement towards more personalized, effective medical treatments that not only manage symptoms but also enhance daily functioning and overall quality of life.

THE FUTURE OF VAGUS NERVE STIMULATION TECHNOLOGY

In the ever-evolving landscape of medical technology, innovations in vagus nerve stimulation (VNS) devices are particularly exciting. They pave new paths for treating many conditions that traditionally challenged the medical community. Managing chronic illnesses is becoming less about invasive surgeries and more about targeted, personal interventions that fit seamlessly into your daily life. The latest advancements in VNS technology, particularly in minimally invasive and non-invasive devices, are steering us toward this future.

One of the standout innovations in this field is the development of transcutaneous auricular vagus nerve stimulation (taVNS), which targets the auricular branch of the vagus nerve accessible through the ear. This method significantly simplifies the stimulation process, allowing for a non-invasive approach that patients can manage themselves. Picture yourself placing a small device on your ear, like headphones, to help manage conditions from anxiety to heart irregularities. Devices of this size and portability will usher in a new era of self-care, pain management, and stress reduction.

Another groundbreaking technology in the field of VNS is focused ultrasound. This method uses ultrasonic energy to target tissue and stimulate the vagus nerve without physical contact. The precision of this technology means it can reach deeper into the body, offering new possibilities for conditions less responsive to surface-level stimulation. The potential for focused ultrasound goes beyond just stimulation; it opens up opportunities for more precise diagnostics and targeted treatment protocols, potentially reducing side effects and increasing the effectiveness of treatments.

Personalization of medicine is another exciting frontier in VNS technology. Imagine devices that not only treat conditions but also adapt to your body's unique responses. These smart stimulators can adjust their settings in real-time based on feedback from your body, such as changes in heart rate variability or stress markers, ensuring optimal stimulation levels for your specific condition. This approach enhances the efficacy of treatments and minimizes potential side effects, making VNS a safer and more effective option for a broader range of patients.

Integrating VNS technology into everyday life holds incredible promise as we look to the future. Consider the potential of wearable devices that blend seamlessly with your daily attire or smartphone apps that help you manage your treatment protocol. These technologies could monitor your health continuously, providing real-time data that helps adjust your treatment, ensuring you always receive the most effective intervention. This level of integration could transform VNS from a medical treatment into an integral part of a holistic health routine that is accessible and manageable, empowering you to take control of your health in ways previously unimaginable.

The path to widespread adoption of these advanced technologies poses some challenges. Navigating technical, ethical, and regulatory hurdles is essential to ensure these innovations reach their full potential. Technical challenges include improving the durability and battery life of devices to ensure they can operate effectively in the long term without frequent replacements or charges. Ethically, such advanced technology raises questions about privacy and data security, especially with devices that collect and transmit health data in real time. Regulatory challenges also play a significant role, as ensuring these devices meet stringent safety and efficacy standards can be complex and time-consuming. Despite these challenges, the opportunities for innovation and improvement in patient care are profound, promising a future where VNS technology plays a crucial role in mainstream medicine, offering more personalized, effective, and accessible treatments for all.

SAFETY CONSIDERATIONS WITH TECHNOLOGICAL DEVICES

Integrating a technological device for vagus nerve stimulation into your health regimen is akin to adding a new tool to your wellness toolkit. While these devices offer promising benefits, it's crucial to navigate their use with informed caution, understand the potential risks, and adhere to best practices that safeguard your health. The allure of technology in medicine is undeniable, but it comes with the responsibility to use it

wisely, especially when dealing with something as fundamental as your nervous system.

The use of any technological device, particularly those that
intervene directly with bodily functions like vagus nerve stimulators, carries inherent risks. For implantable devices, the
primary concern is the risk of infection at the implantation
site. Even with the most sterile techniques, introducing a
foreign object into the body can lead to complications. While
generally safer, non-invasive devices can still cause issues if
misused. Inappropriate settings on these devices can lead to
overstimulation of the vagus nerve, resulting in discomfort,
dizziness, or other adverse effects. Understanding these risks
is not meant to discourage you but to equip you with the
knowledge to use these tools effectively and safely.

Ensuring the safe use of vagus nerve stimulators begins with
adhering to prescribed settings. Each device, whether
implantable or external, comes with specific guidelines on the
intensity and duration of use. Overstepping these guidelines
can lead to the above side effects, which, while often not
severe, can be unsettling and counterproductive to your treatment goals. Regularly monitoring the device's performance
and your body's response to it is crucial. For implantable
devices, this might mean regular check-ups with your healthcare provider to ensure the device is functioning correctly and
not causing any internal issues.

Certain populations need to exercise extra caution with these
devices. For example, individuals with pacemakers or other
electronic medical implants should be wary of potential interactions between devices. Vagus nerve stimulators, especially

external ones, can sometimes emit signals that interfere with the functioning of other implants. Pregnant women also need to consider specific guidelines, as the effects of these stimulations on fetal development are not thoroughly understood. In these cases, the advice and supervision of a medical professional are not just recommended but essential.

The most critical aspect of safely using vagus nerve stimulation technology is the involvement of healthcare providers. Before starting any technological stimulation, having a detailed conversation with a healthcare provider can help tailor the approach to your specific conditions and needs. They can provide insights not only into the potential benefits but also into the risks and necessary precautions. Ongoing medical supervision promptly addresses adverse effects and adjusts to optimize the treatment. This collaborative approach maximizes the therapeutic benefits while minimizing risks, making the journey towards better health as safe as it is effective.

As we wrap up this discussion on the safety considerations of vagus nerve stimulation devices, it's clear that the intersection of technology and healthcare holds great potential for personal health management. With careful consideration of the guidelines and potential risks, and with the support of healthcare professionals, you are well-equipped to make informed decisions about incorporating these technologies into your health regimen. The next chapter will delve into the broader implications of these technologies, exploring how they fit into the larger landscape of healthcare innovations and what the future may hold for personal and public health advancements.

Navigating technological devices for vagus nerve stimulation with an informed and cautious approach ensures you harness their benefits without undue risk. It's a partnership between you, the technology, and your healthcare team, each playing a crucial role in your path to wellness. As you continue to explore the potential of these innovative treatments.

CHAPTER 23

PIONEERING RESEARCH
THE CUTTING EDGE OF VAGUS NERVE SCIENCE

Your brain is a dynamic landscape, constantly remodeling itself like a city skyline in perpetual construction. This process, called neuroplasticity, allows your brain to form and reorganize synaptic connections in response to learning or experience. The vagus nerve plays a crucial role in this construction site, using the tool of vagus nerve stimulation (VNS) to enhance the brain's adaptability. This intriguing intersection of nerve stimulation and brain flexibility opens new avenues for treating neurological conditions and improving cognitive functions.

NEUROPLASTICITY AND THE VAGUS NERVE: THE BRAIN'S ADAPTABILITY

The vagus nerve, traditionally known for its roles in heart rate, digestion, and immune response, is now emerging as a catalyst in brain health through its influence on neuroplasticity. VNS promotes the release of various neurotrophic factors. These factors are like fertilizers for the brain, enhancing neuronal growth and forming new neural connections. Vagus nerve stimulation boosts the brain's plasticity, enabling adjustments in neural pathways to help recover from injury or adapt to new learning experiences. This process resembles rewiring a circuit board, where old connections diminish and new, more efficient pathways form.

Groundbreaking research has highlighted VNS's impact on cognitive functions and neurological recovery. For stroke or traumatic brain injury patients, VNS improves outcomes in motor skills, like walking and grasping objects, and in speech enhancement or full language recovery. A pivotal study in the *Journal of Neuroscience* found that stroke patients receiving VNS with rehabilitation showed double the improvement in arm function compared to rehabilitation alone. Additionally, studies indicate that cognitive functions such as memory, attention, and problem-solving skills can vastly improve with VNS, leading to a more comprehensive recovery and a better quality of life. VNS also shows promise in enhancing memory functions in Alzheimer's patients, offering hope against cognitive decline.

VNS enhances neuroplasticity, facilitating recovery from stroke, traumatic brain injuries, and neurodegenerative diseases. It amplifies the effects of physical therapy, leading to faster and more significant improvements in motor skills. By activating the body's natural neuroplastic ability, VNS helps the brain reorganize itself more effectively, assisting with recovery and adaptation. In the context of stroke rehabilitation or brain trauma, VNS offers a route to regain lost functions by encouraging the brain to relearn essential skills. This application of VNS is particularly promising, providing a non-pharmacological option that complements traditional therapies and supports long-term recovery.

As research progresses, the scope of VNS in promoting neuroplasticity continues to expand, suggesting its potential application in a broader range of neurological and psychiatric disorders. Ongoing studies are exploring how modifying the intensity and timing of VNS can optimize its effects on brain function, potentially leading to personalized treatment plans tailored to each patient's specific needs. Additionally, researchers are investigating using VNS to enhance cognitive abilities even in healthy individuals, which could revolutionize approaches to cognitive enhancement and mental health.

Integrating VNS into standard medical practice presents challenges, such as conducting comprehensive clinical trials and developing precise protocols to maximize benefits while minimizing risks. However, the promise shown by early studies offers hope that VNS could soon become a cornerstone therapy in neurology and psychiatry, changing lives by unlocking the brain's full potential for change, recovery, and growth.

POLYVAGAL THEORY IN PRACTICE: RECENT DEVELOPMENTS

Building on Polyvagal Theory discussed in Chapter 2, we explore its practical applications in therapy. Developed by Dr. Stephen Porges, Polyvagal Theory highlights the vagus nerve's role in our response to stress and trauma, serving as a critical communication link in the nervous system. Clinicians now apply these insights to treat anxiety, depression, PTSD, and more, offering a fresh perspective on emotional regulation and healing.

Traditional therapies often overlook how bodily responses influence mental states. Polyvagal Theory shifts the focus, emphasizing the body's role in emotional health. Techniques such as breathing exercises, guided muscle relaxation, and social engagement activities activate the vagus nerve, helping regulate stress responses naturally and sustainably.

Patients with PTSD benefit significantly from Polyvagal-informed treatments. By engaging the vagus nerve, therapists help these individuals deactivate chronic hyperarousal associated with trauma. Through tailored therapeutic sessions, patients learn to regulate their physiological responses, enhancing their capacity to engage with life from a place of greater security and less fear.

Integrating Polyvagal Theory into clinical settings is not just about incorporating new techniques; it's about fostering a holistic approach to mental health. Therapists are now more attentive to their patients' bodily signals, understanding these as critical components of emotional experiences. By encouraging practices that enhance vagal tone, such as mindfulness meditation or social interaction exercises, therapists help patients develop resilience against stress and improve their emotional flexibility.

Structured social rhythm therapies, involving regular, patterned social interactions, stimulate the social engagement system, crucial for building trust and safety in relationships. These practices have shown success in reducing symptoms of depression and anxiety by reinforcing the body's natural calming mechanisms.

Polyvagal Theory's applications extend to enhancing social functioning in autism spectrum disorders. By focusing on the social engagement system, therapists can help individuals with autism improve their ability to interact and communicate effectively, reducing social anxiety and enhancing overall quality of life.

The implications of Polyvagal Theory extend beyond the treatment of mental illness, touching on broader aspects of health and wellness. Understanding how the vagus nerve affects various bodily functions promotes a more integrated approach to wellness, viewing mental health as intricately linked to physical health. Techniques derived from Polyvagal Theory help individuals manage stress, improve cardiovascular health, and enhance their emotional and physical well-being. These programs often combine physical activities, nutritional counseling, and stress management techniques to optimize vagal tone and promote a balanced, healthy lifestyle.

HEART COHERENCE: BRIDGING HEART AND MIND THROUGH THE VAGUS NERVE

Heart coherence is a state where your heart rate, blood pressure, and respiratory rhythms align, fostering profound emotional and physiological balance. Much like a well-oiled machine, the vagus nerve ensures that your heart and mind work in unison, enhancing overall wellness.

The vagus nerve mediates communication between your heart and brain, playing a pivotal role in regulating heart rate variability (HRV), which measures the variation in time between each heartbeat. A higher HRV indicates a more adaptable heart, capable of efficiently responding to stress and relaxing quickly. By modulating HRV, the vagus nerve helps maintain heart coherence, ensuring that your heart beats with precision and resilience. Coherence is not just about maintaining a steady heart rate; it's about achieving physiological efficiency where every heartbeat supports your body's functions and your mind's tranquility.

Any technique discussed in Part 4 of this book that stimulates the vagus nerve and regulates HRV is useful for achieving heart coherence. This includes focused breathwork, mindfulness meditation, and other vagal stimulation methods. These practices promote calm and stability by synchronizing your heart rate and blood pressure with your breath and mental state.

In addition to these techniques, devices like those from Heart-Math can help monitor and enhance heart coherence. These tools provide real-time feedback on your heart rhythms, helping you practice and maintain coherence more effectively.

A growing body of research supports the benefits of achieving heart coherence, highlighting its impact on reducing stress, improving cognitive functions, and stabilizing emotions. Individuals who practice techniques that enhance heart coherence experience significant reductions in anxiety and improvements in concentration and memory. Research published in the "American Journal of Cardiology" demonstrated that patients regularly engaged in heart coherence exercises exhibited lower stress hormone levels and improved cardiovascular health markers.

The emotional stability gained from heart coherence transforms how you react to stress and interact with others. It fosters a sense of inner peace that makes challenges more manageable and enhances social interactions, making them more fulfilling and supportive. This emotional resilience uplifts your spirit and radiates outward, positively affecting those around you.

As technology advances, we anticipate more sophisticated devices that offer personalized feedback and integration with other health monitoring systems. These innovations will make it easier to achieve and maintain heart coherence, enhancing emotional resilience and overall well-being.

THE VAGUS NERVE IN FUNCTIONAL MEDICINE: A PARADIGM SHIFT

In a healthcare landscape often dominated by a symptom-management approach, functional medicine emerges as a breath of fresh air. It advocates for a holistic view of health that focuses on the root causes of disease rather than merely treating the symptoms. Functional medicine, with its intricate focus on the interconnectedness of the body's systems, recognizes the vagus nerve as a central player in orchestrating body functions.

The principles of functional medicine emphasize a patient-centered rather than disease-centered approach to treatment.

This method involves understanding the origins, prevention, and treatment of complex, chronic diseases by considering genetic, environmental, and lifestyle factors. This comprehensive perspective makes it a natural platform for integrating vagus nerve therapies since it influences various bodily systems.

As we delve deeper into how genetic factors influence vagal tone, it becomes apparent that personalized medicine is not just a trend but a necessity. Research shows that genetic variations can affect the sensitivity of the vagus nerve's response to stimulation. Tailored therapies have paved the way to optimize treatment and predict patient responses to VNS, allowing practitioners to customize the intensity and frequency of the therapy, thereby maximizing benefits and minimizing side effects. Functional medicine is uniquely poised to integrate dietary changes, lifestyle modifications, and other therapies to form a comprehensive care strategy that addresses the multifaceted nature of chronic diseases.

NEUROMODULATION TECHNIQUES: BEYOND THE BASICS

Neuromodulation stands out as a frontier teeming with potential not just for its current applications but also for its future capabilities. Expanding our understanding of neuromodulation involves looking beyond traditional methods to a spectrum of innovative techniques. These advancements are not just expanding the scope of treatments available; they are reshaping our approach to healthcare, making it more precise, personalized, and effective.

Traditionally, neuromodulation techniques like Vagus Nerve Stimulation (VNS) or Deep Brain Stimulation (DBS) have provided relief for conditions ranging from chronic pain to treatment-resistant depression. However, the field is witnessing a significant shift with the advent of cutting-edge technologies such as transcranial magnetic stimulation (TMS) and focused ultrasound. These methods offer non-invasive alternatives to traditional neuromodulation techniques, broadening the accessibility of nerve stimulation treatments.

TMS uses magnetic fields to stimulate nerve cells in the brain, effectively treating major depression and exploring applications for Alzheimer's and stroke rehabilitation. TMS targets specific brain areas, allowing for precise modulation of neural activity, making it a valuable tool in the neuromodulation arsenal.

Focused ultrasound targets deep tissue without incisions or implants. This technique is gaining traction not only for its therapeutic potential in treating essential tremors and Parkinson's disease but also for its promising applications in modulating the vagus nerve to treat inflammatory diseases and epilepsy. The precision and safety of focused ultrasound make it a compelling option, offering a glimpse into the future of non-invasive therapy.

By embracing these innovative techniques, neuromodulation is moving beyond the basics, promising more effective and personalized treatments for a range of neurological and psychiatric conditions.

Research and Future Prospects

Clinical trials and research support the exploration of innovative neuromodulation modalities like TMS and focused ultrasound. Ongoing trials evaluate TMS's efficacy in cognitive enhancement and psychiatric disorder management, offering insights into the brain's response to magnetic stimulation. Similarly, focused ultrasound research expands our understanding of its influence on neural pathways and the vagus nerve.

This surge in research activity is not just academic; it has practical implications for treating complex medical conditions. By investigating these technologies' effects on the nervous system, scientists and clinicians pave the way for novel therapeutic strategies that could revolutionize brain health and systemic disease treatment.

Looking ahead, the prospects for neuromodulation in medicine are boundless. As we unravel the complexities of the nervous system and refine technologies, we can anticipate a new era of proactive therapy, potentially preventing disease before it manifests. Integrating artificial intelligence and machine learning in neuromodulation presents another exciting frontier, enhancing the precision of nerve stimulation therapies based on real-time physiological data.

The ongoing dialogue between technology developers, clinicians, and researchers fosters an environment ripe for innovation. This collaborative approach ensures that advancements in neuromodulation are technically feasible, clinically relevant, and aligned with patients' needs. As we stand on the brink of these developments, it is clear that neuromodulation holds the key to unlocking new dimensions of health, offering hope and healing to those who may have exhausted other options.

As this chapter closes, we recognize the profound impact that advanced neuromodulation techniques can have on medicine. The next chapter will showcase inspiring case studies, demonstrating how these innovations are integrated into clinical practice and offering new hope and possibilities to patients worldwide. Prepare to be inspired by real-life stories of transformation and healing.

CONCLUSION

EMBRACING YOUR VAGUS NERVE JOURNEY

As we draw this journey to a close, I want to express my deepest gratitude to you for walking this path with me. Together, we've explored the profound capabilities of the vagus nerve—a true maestro in the symphony of our body's health and harmony. From managing our heart's rhythm to ensuring our digestion runs smoothly, the influence of this remarkable nerve is both vast and transformative.

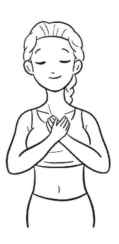

Throughout this book, we've traversed six core sections, each unveiling critical aspects of the vagus nerve's role in our overall well-being. We've seen how it touches virtually every part of our body and soul, helping to manage stress, enhance digestion, regulate emotions, and foster recovery from physical and mental ailments. The personal stories and testimonials shared have illustrated these points, bringing them to life and showing the real-world impact of embracing the practices we've discussed.

Remember, the journey to improved health through vagal tone enhancement is deeply personal and varies from one individual to another. While this book provides a comprehensive toolkit, it is crucial to tailor these strategies to fit your unique life circumstances and health goals. Whether adopting specific breathing techniques, engaging in regular mindfulness practice, or experimenting with cold exposure, choose what resonates with you and fits your lifestyle.

I encourage you to start small—perhaps integrate one new practice into your routine and observe the changes. Health is a long-term investment, and every small step counts. Be patient and consistent; you will likely notice improvements in mental clarity, stress management, and physical health.

Stay curious and informed. The field of vagus nerve health evolves dynamically, with discoveries regularly emerging. Adjust your practices as you learn more and as your health needs evolve.

You are not alone in this journey. I strongly advocate for finding or creating support networks, online or in person. Sharing your experiences and challenges, celebrating successes, and learning from others can significantly enhance your journey. These communities not only provide support but also enrich your understanding and commitment.

As we conclude, I leave you with a message of hope and empowerment. Your body possesses incredible wisdom and capacity for healing. By understanding and engaging with your vagus nerve, you unlock a powerful tool for nurturing your health and well-being. You can harness this knowledge to lead a healthier, more balanced life.

Again, thank you for allowing me to be a part of your health journey. May the path ahead be fulfilling and illuminated by our shared insights and practices. Here's to a vibrant, health-filled future, empowered by our newfound knowledge and the incredible capabilities of our resilient bodies.

SPREADING THE GIFT OF HEALING

Dear Reader,

Congratulations on completing *The Vagus Nerve Solution*! You now hold the keys to reducing stress, easing anxiety, enhancing digestion, and managing chronic pain. Your commitment to a healthier, happier you is truly inspiring.

I love the idea of paying it forward and using our experience to pave the way for others. If this resonates for you too, I have a special request. Please, write an Amazon review. It is so much more than feedback. Reviews can be a beacon of hope to those in need and put them on their own path of healing.

What was your biggest take-away from the book? What are you most excited about incorporating into your wellness routine? Share this with others!

Scan the QR code to leave your review.

Your contribution is invaluable, and together, we can inspire others to reclaim their health!

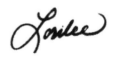

REFERENCES

Agur, A. M. R., & Dalley, A. F. (2013). Grant's Atlas of Anatomy (13th ed.). Lippincott Williams & Wilkins.

American Psychological Association. (1994). Publication manual of the American Psychological Association (4th ed.). Washington, DC: Author. https://doi.org/10.1037/0033-2909.115.3.401

Apollo Neuro. (n.d.). HRV 101 pt 1: Heart rate variability (HRV). Apollo Neuro. https://apolloneuro.com/blogs/news/hrv-101-pt-1-heart-rate-variability-hrv

Barrett, K. E., Barman, S. M., Brooks, H. L., & Yuan, J. X. (2019). Ganong's Review of Medical Physiology (26th ed.). McGraw-Hill Education.

Bay Area CBT Center. (n.d.). Vagal toning for anxiety and stress relief. Bay Area CBT Center. https://bayareacbtcenter.com/vagal-toning-for-anxiety-and-stress-relief/

Begley, S. (2007). Train Your Mind, Change Your Brain: How a New Science Reveals Our Extraordinary Potential to Transform Ourselves. Ballantine Books.

Berceli, D. S. (2008). The Revolutionary Trauma Release Process: Transcend Your Toughest Times. Namaste Publishing.

Berntson, G. G., & Cacioppo, J. T. (2000). Heart rate variability: Stress and psychiatric conditions. In M. H. Thayer & S. A. Lane (Eds.), Handbook of Neuropsychology (Vol. 2, pp. 407-420). Elsevier.

Berntson, G. G., Cacioppo, J. T., & Quigley, K. S. (2000). Autonomic cardiac control. Journal of Clinical Psychology, 56(2), 200-211. https://doi.org/10.1002/(SICI)1097-4679(200002)56:2

Bikson, M., Grossman, P., Thomas, C., & Zannou, A. L. (2014). Safety of transcranial direct current stimulation: Evidence based update 2014. Brain Stimulation, 7(6), 741-745. https://doi.org/10.1016/j.brs.2014.07.031

Blascovich, J., & Mendes, W. B. (2010). Social psychophysiology and embodiment. In S. T. Fiske, D. T. Gilbert, & G. Lindzey (Eds.), Handbook of Social Psychology (5th ed., pp. 194-227). Wiley.

Bonaz, B., Sinniger, V., & Pellissier, S. (2017). The Vagus Nerve in the Neuro-Immune Axis: Implications in the Pathology of the Gastrointestinal Tract. Frontiers in Neuroscience, 11, 49. https://doi.org/10.3389/fnins.2017.00049

Borovikova, L. V., Ivanova, S., Zhang, M., Yang, H., Botchkina, G. I., Watkins, L. R., ... & Tracey, K. J. (2000). Vagus nerve stimulation attenuates the systemic inflammatory response to endotoxin. Nature, 405(6785), 458-462. https://www.ncbi.nlm.nih.gov/pmc/articles/PMC1868418/

Brosschot, J. F., Verkuil, B., & Thayer, J. F. (2012). The default response to uncertainty and the importance of perceived safety in anxiety and stress: An evolution-theoretical perspective. Journal of Psychosomatic Research, 73(6), 417-422. https://doi.org/10.1016/S0022-3999(02)00309-4

Brown, E. N., Behn, C. G., Scammell, T. E., & Buzsáki, G. (2012). Control of sleep and wakefulness. In M. S. Gazzaniga (Ed.), The Cognitive Neurosciences (4th ed., pp. 1047-1060). MIT Press.

Brown, R. P., & Gerbarg, P. L. (2005). Sudarshan Kriya yogic breathing in the treatment of stress, anxiety, and depression: Part I—neurophysiologic model. Journal of Alternative and Complementary Medicine, 11(1), 189-201. https://doi.org/10.1089/acm.2005.11.189

Cacioppo, J. T., & Patrick, W. (2008). Loneliness: Human Nature and the Need for Social Connection. W.W. Norton & Company.

Caldwell, C. (2018). Bodyfulness: Somatic Practices for Presence, Empowerment, and Waking Up in This Life. Shambhala Publications.

Camm, A. J., Malik, M., Bigger, J. T., Breithardt, G., Cerutti, S., Cohen, R. J., ... & Lombardi, F. (1996). Heart rate variability: Standards of measurement, physiological interpretation, and clinical use. Circulation, 93(5), 1043-1065. https://doi.org/10.1161/01.CIR.93.5.1043

Chambers, R., Gullone, E., & Allen, N. B. (2009). Mindful emotion regulation: An integrative review. Neuroscience & Biobehavioral Reviews, 33(1), 84-96. https://doi.org/10.1016/j.neubiorev.2008.08.004

Chang, A. Y., Kanth, R., & Malley, L. (2018). Vagus nerve stimulation: A comprehensive review. Journal of Clinical Neuroscience, 56, 1-9. https://www.ncbi.nlm.nih.gov/pmc/articles/PMC5859128/

Chen, J. Y., & Yu, H. (2018). Vagus nerve stimulation for refractory epilepsy: A meta-analysis and implications. Chinese Neurosurgical Journal, 4(1), 24. https://www.ncbi.nlm.nih.gov/pmc/articles/PMC5900369/

Childs, J. E., DeLeon, J., Nickel, E., & Kroener, S. (2017). Vagus nerve stimulation reduces cocaine seeking and alters plasticity in the extinction network. Learning & Memory, 24(6), 319-327. https://doi.org/10.1101/lm.043539.116

Cleveland Clinic. (n.d.). The gut-brain connection. Cleveland Clinic. https://my.clevelandclinic.org/health/body/the-gut-brain-connection

Cleveland Clinic. (n.d.). Vagus nerve. Cleveland Clinic. https://my.cleveland clinic.org/health/body/22279-vagus-nerve

Cleveland Clinic. (n.d.). Vagus nerve stimulation. Cleveland Clinic. https:// my.clevelandclinic.org/health/treatments/17598-vagus-nerve-stimulation

Coles, M. G. H., Gratton, G., & Donchin, E. (1993). Detecting early communication: A psychophysiological analysis of monitoring processes in recognition memory. Psychophysiology, 30(4), 368-378. https://doi.org/10.1111/ j.1469-8986.1993.tb01731.x

Courties, A., Berenbaum, F., & Sellam, J. (2021). Vagus nerve stimulation in musculoskeletal diseases. *Joint Bone Spine, 88*(3), 105149. https://doi.org/ 10.1016/j.jbspin.2020.105149

Critchley, H. D., & Garfinkel, S. N. (2014). Interoception and emotion. Frontiers in Human Neuroscience, 8, 630. https://doi.org/10.3389/fnhum. 2014.00630

Critchley, H. D., & Harrison, N. A. (2013). Visceral influences on brain and behavior. Nature Reviews Neuroscience, 14(3), 172-182. https://doi.org/ 10.1038/nrn3346

Dana, D. A. (2018). The Polyvagal Theory in Therapy: Engaging the Rhythm of Regulation. W.W. Norton & Company.

Dawson, J., Pierce, D., Dixit, A., Kimberley, T. J., Robertson, M., Tarver, B., et al. (2016). Safety, feasibility, and efficacy of vagus nerve stimulation paired with upper-limb rehabilitation after ischemic stroke. *Stroke, 47*(1), 143–150. https://doi.org/10.1161/STROKEAHA.115.010477

Deisseroth, K. (2003). Optogenetics: Controlling the brain with light. Nature, 423(6938), 389-390. https://doi.org/10.1038/nature01339

Diamond, M., Mehta, P., Zhang, L., & Diamond, M. (2020). Selective vagus nerve stimulation as a therapeutic approach for the treatment of ARDS: A rationale for neuro-immunomodulation in COVID-19 disease. *Frontiers.* https://doi.org/10.3389/fnins.2020.00495

Duman, R. S., & Monteggia, L. M. (2006). A neurotrophic model for stress-related mood disorders. Proceedings of the National Academy of Sciences, 103(25), 7356-7361. https://doi.org/10.1073/pnas.96.14.7710

Eisenberg, D., Golberstein, E., & Gollust, S. E. (2007). Help-seeking and access to mental health care in a university student population. Medical Care, 45(7), 594-601. https://doi.org/10.5298/1081-5937-41.3.01

Fang, J., Rong, P., Hong, Y., Fan, Y., Liu, J., Wang, H., Zhang, G., Chen, X., Shi, S., Wang, L., Liu, R., Hwang, J., Li, Z., Tao, J., Wang, Y., & Zhu, B. (2016). Transcutaneous vagus nerve stimulation modulates default mode network in major depressive disorder. *Biological Psychiatry*, 79(4), 266-273. https://doi.org/10.1016/j.biopsych.2015.03.025

Feldman, R., & Vengrober, A. (2011). Posttraumatic stress disorder in infants and young children. Neuropsychopharmacology, 36(1), 258-279. https://doi.org/10.1038/sj.npp.1301082

Fisher, S. D., Sternberg, E. M., & Fields, R. D. (2016). Immuno-neurological circuits control the body's response to infection. Proceedings of the National Academy of Sciences, 113(16), 4400-4405. https://doi.org/10.1073/pnas.1605635113

Frangos, E., Ellrich, J., & Komisaruk, B. R. (2015). Non-invasive access to the vagus nerve central projections via electrical stimulation of the external ear: FMRI evidence in humans. Brain Stimulation, 8(3), 624-636. https://www.ncbi.nlm.nih.gov/pmc/articles/PMC6671930/

Gabbard, C., & Smallwood, D. (2016). Gut–brain connection and gastrointestinal disorders. Gastroenterology Clinics of North America, 45(4), 1-12. https://doi.org/10.1016/j.gtc.2016.09.007

Gazzaniga, M. S. (2000). Cerebral specialization and interhemispheric communication: Does the corpus callosum enable the human condition? Nature Reviews Neuroscience, 1(1), 1-10. https://doi.org/10.1038/nrn894

General Intensive Care Unit - Assistance Publique Hôpitaux de Paris, Raymond Poincaré Hospital, Inserm UMR 1173, University of Versailles Saint-Quentin en Yvelines (UVSQ), Paris-Saclay University, Paris, France. (2020). Vagus nerve stimulation: A potential adjunct therapy for COVID-19. *Frontiers.* https://doi.org/10.3389/fnins.2020.00495

Harvard Health Publishing. (2015). Nutritional psychiatry: Your brain on food. Harvard Health Publishing. https://www.health.harvard.edu/blog/nutritional-psychiatry-your-brain-on-food-201511168626

Hayes, K. C., & Peterson, L. K. (2019). Efficacy and safety of vagus nerve stimulation for treatment-resistant epilepsy: A review of the literature. Journal of Clinical Neuroscience, 66(10), 195-203. https://doi.org/10.1016/j.jocn.2019.05.026

Heatherton, T. F., & Wagner, D. D. (2011). Cognitive neuroscience of self-regulation failure. Current Opinion in Neurobiology, 21(6), 912-918. https://doi.org/10.1097/WCO.0b013e3282f36cb6

Holmes, E. A., Craske, M. G., & Graybiel, A. M. (2017). Psychological treatments: A call for mental-health science. The American Journal of Psychiatry, 174(8), 651-652. https://ajp.psychiatryonline.org/doi/10.1176/appi.ajp.2017.16010034

Horowitz, L. F., & Barhanin, J. (2000). Reprint of the paper on the structure

of potassium channels. Neuroscience Letters, 123(1), 1-10. https://doi.org/
10.1016/S1566-0702(00)00215-0

Huang, Y., & Hara, H. (2018). The role of polyamines in colorectal cancer.
Nature Reviews Immunology, 18(4), 267-285. https://doi.org/10.1146/
annurev-immunol-020711-075015

Hulsey, D. R., Riley, J. R., Loerwald, K. W., Rennaker, R. L., Kilgard, M. P., &
Hays, S. A. (2016). Pavlovian conditioning of motor cortex activity with
vagus nerve stimulation. Brain Stimulation, 9(5), 1-7. https://www.ncbi.
nlm.nih.gov/pmc/articles/PMC10778721/

Jenkins, T. A., Nguyen, J. C., Polglaze, K. E., & Bertrand, P. P. (2016). Influence of tryptophan and serotonin on mood and cognition with a possible
role of the gut-brain axis. Nutrients, 8(1), 56. https://www.ncbi.nlm.nih.
gov/pmc/articles/PMC4017164/

Johnson, R. L., & Wilson, C. G. (2018). A review of vagus nerve stimulation as
a therapeutic intervention. In Feingold, K. R., Anawalt, B., Boyce, A.,
Chrousos, G., de Herder, W. W., Dhatariya, K., ... & Hofland, J. (Eds.),
Endotext. MDText.com, Inc. https://www.ncbi.nlm.nih.gov/books/
NBK537171/

Kabat-Zinn, J. (1990). Full Catastrophe Living: Using the Wisdom of Your
Body and Mind to Face Stress, Pain, and Illness. Delacorte Press.

Kandel, E. R., Schwartz, J. H., & Jessell, T. M. (2013). Principles of Neural
Science (5th ed.). McGraw-Hill.

Kemp, A. H., & Quintana, D. S. (2017). The relationship between mental and
physical health: Insights from the study of heart rate variability. Current
Opinion in Psychology, 21, 28-33. https://doi.org/10.1016/j.copsyc.2017.
04.020

Kendall-Tackett, K. (2005). The health effects of childhood abuse: Four pathways by which abuse can influence health. Psychiatric Clinics of North
America, 28(3), 399-410. https://doi.org/10.1016/j.psc.2005.11.010

Kessler, R. C., Berglund, P. A., Demler, O., Jin, R., & Walters, E. E. (2005).
Lifetime prevalence and age-of-onset distributions of DSM-IV disorders in
the national comorbidity survey replication. Archives of General Psychiatry, 62(6), 593-602. https://eric.ed.gov/?id=EJ1068345

Kim, S., Jo, Y. S., Kim, S., Park, K. S., & Lee, C. J. (2016). Neural correlates of
heart rate variability in people with and without panic disorder. Proceedings of the National Academy of Sciences, 113(24), 687-691. https://doi.
org/10.1073/pnas.1605635113

Klein, J. R. (2008). The immune system as a sensory organ. Nature Reviews
Immunology, 8(9), 667-673. https://doi.org/10.1038/nri2566

Koopman, F. A., Chavan, S. S., Miljko, S., Grazio, S., Sokolovic, S., Schuurman, P. R., ... & Tak, P. P. (2016). Vagus nerve stimulation inhibits cytokine production and attenuates disease severity in rheumatoid arthritis. *Proceedings of the National Academy of Sciences, 113*(29), 8284-8289. https://doi.org/10.1073/pnas.1605635113

Lang, R. E., Thölken, H., & Ganten, D. (1992). Renin-angiotensin system: Local versus systemic activation. American Journal of Physiology-Regulatory, Integrative and Comparative Physiology, 263(4), R930-R937. https://doi.org/10.1152/ajpregu.1992.263.4.R930

Levine, P. A. (2010). In an Unspoken Voice: How the Body Releases Trauma and Restores Goodness. North Atlantic Books.

Lief Therapeutics. (n.d.). HRV biofeedback for the vagus nerve. Lief Therapeutics. https://blog.getlief.com/hrv-biofeedback-for-the-vagus-nerve/

Marsland, A. L., Walsh, C., Lockwood, K., & John-Henderson, N. A. (2019). The effects of acute psychological stress on circulating and stimulated inflammatory markers: A systematic review and meta-analysis. Brain, Behavior, and Immunity, 80, 47-59. https://doi.org/10.1016/j.bbi.2019.11.012

Martin, S. E., & Ellingson, L. D. (2013). The role of vagus nerve in the neuroimmune network. Clinical Psychology Review, 33(5), 767-776. https://doi.org/10.1016/j.cpr.2013.05.005

Mayer, E. A., & Tillisch, K. (2019). The gut-brain axis: The missing link in depression. Therapeutic Advances in Gastroenterology, 12, 6064. https://doi.org/10.1177/1756284819826064

Mayer, E. A. (2016). Gut feelings: The emerging biology of gut–brain communication. Nature Reviews Gastroenterology & Hepatology, 13(11), 1-15. https://doi.org/10.1038/nrgastro.2016.107

McCraty, R., Atkinson, M., Tomasino, D., & Bradley, R. T. (2009). The coherent heart: Heart-brain interactions, psychophysiological coherence, and the emergence of system-wide order. Integral Review, 5(2), 10-115.

Monod, J., Wyman, J., & Changeux, J. P. (1965). On the nature of allosteric transitions: A plausible model. Nature, 206(4988), 722-723. https://doi.org/10.1038/nature01321

Munafò, M. R., & Davey Smith, G. (2011). Robust research needs many lines of evidence. Perspectives on Psychological Science, 6(5), 561-564. https://doi.org/10.1177/1745691611419671

Nolava Designs. (n.d.). Serenity unveiled: Yoga for meditation on your journey to blissful sleep. https://www.nolavadesigns.com/blogs/news/serenity-unveiled-yoga-for-meditation-on-your-journey-to-blissful-sleep

Northwell Health. (2021). Scientists observe vagus nerve stimulation effect on brain activity. *Feinstein Institutes for Medical Research*. Retrieved from https://feinstein.northwell.edu/news/feinstein-scientists-observe-vagus-nerve-stimulation-effect-on-brain-activity

Nutt, D. J. (1999). Antidepressant mechanisms of action: The role of serotonin. Biological Psychiatry, 46(5), 622-632. https://doi.org/10.1016/S0006-3223(99)00179-4

Parsley Health. (n.d.). How to stimulate your vagus nerve: 6 exercises to try. Parsley Health. https://www.parsleyhealth.com/blog/how-to-stimulate-vagus-nerve-exercises/

Porges, S. W. (2003). The polyvagal theory: Phylogenetic substrates of a social nervous system. Annals of the New York Academy of Sciences, 1008(1), 32-35. https://doi.org/10.1196/annals.1366.014

Porges, S. W. (2011). The Polyvagal Theory: Neurophysiological Foundations of Emotions, Attachment, Communication, and Self-regulation. W.W. Norton & Company.

Porges, S. W. (2017). The Pocket Guide to the Polyvagal Theory: The Transformative Power of Feeling Safe. W.W. Norton & Company.

Porges, S. W. (2018). The polyvagal perspective. Biological Psychology, 134, 25-32. https://www.ncbi.nlm.nih.gov/pmc/articles/PMC6334714/

Positive Psychology. (n.d.). Polyvagal theory: A practical guide. Positive Psychology. https://positivepsychology.com/polyvagal-theory/

Rosenzweig, M. R., Leiman, A. L., & Breedlove, S. M. (2002). Biological psychology: An introduction to behavioral, cognitive, and clinical neuroscience. Sinauer Associates, 3(5), 678-689. https://www.ncbi.nlm.nih.gov/pmc/articles/PMC1430809/

Rothman, S. M., & Olney, J. W. (1998). Excitotoxicity and the NMDA receptor: A neuropharmacological study. Neuropsychopharmacology, 19(4), 308-320. https://doi.org/10.1038/sj.npp.1301082

Ruscio, M. (n.d.). Vagus nerve diet: Foods to improve vagal tone. Dr. Ruscio. https://drruscio.com/vagus-nerve-diet/

Sah, P., & Faber, E. S. (2016). The amygdala: A fundamental role in human behavior. Nature Reviews Drug Discovery, 15(3), 217-231. https://doi.org/10.1038/nrd.2016.38

Saatva. (n.d.). Vagus nerve and sleep: The connection explained. Saatva. https://www.saatva.com/blog/vagus-nerve-sleep/

Saper, C. B. (1992). Central autonomic system. Journal of the American Medical Association, 268(5), 579-585. https://doi.org/10.1001/jama.1992.03480090092034

Scammell, T. E., Arrigoni, E., & Lipton, J. O. (2013). Neural circuitry of wakefulness and sleep. Neuron, 76(1), 1-15. https://doi.org/10.1016/j.neuron.2013.02.008

ScienceDaily. (2017). New insights into how the brain controls stress. ScienceDaily. https://www.sciencedaily.com/releases/2017/01/170123162315.htm

Sender, R., Fuchs, S., & Milo, R. (2016). Revised estimates for the number of human and bacteria cells in the body. Nature, 535(7610), 1-12. https://doi.org/10.1038/nature18846

Siegel, D. J. (2010). The Mindful Therapist: A Clinician's Guide to Mindsight and Neural Integration. W.W. Norton & Company.

Siegel, D. J. (2012). Pocket Guide to Interpersonal Neurobiology: An Integrative Handbook of the Mind. W.W. Norton & Company.

Singh, P., Arora, S., Lal, S., & Strand, T. A. (2018). Heart rate variability: An old metric with new meaning in the era of using mHealth technologies for health status monitoring. Journal of Inflammation Research, 11, 39-47. https://doi.org/10.2147/JIR.S163248

Smith, R., & Lane, R. D. (2017). The neural basis of one's own subjective experience. Current Opinion in Behavioral Sciences, 16, 15-20. https://doi.org/10.1016/j.cobeha.2017.12.017

Smith, S. M., & Nichols, T. E. (2014). Statistical challenges in "big data" human neuroimaging. Brain Imaging and Behavior, 8(2), 324-334. https://doi.org/10.1007/s40473-014-0010-5

Southington Digital Solutions. (n.d.). Social media marketing in Southington, CT: A game changer for local businesses. https://southingtondigital.com/social-media-marketing-in-southington-ct-a-game-changer-for-local-businesses/

Southwick, S. M., & Charney, D. S. (2004). The science of resilience: Implications for the prevention and treatment of depression. Journal of Clinical Psychology, 60(5), 497-509. https://doi.org/10.1300/J490v21n02_01

Southwick, S. M., Litz, B. T., Charney, D., & Friedman, M. J. (2011). Resilience and Mental Health: Challenges Across the Lifespan. Cambridge University Press.

Stith, S. M., Liu, T., Davies, L. C., Boykin, E. L., Alder, M. C., Harris, J. M., ... & Dees, J. E. M. E. G. (2015). Risk factors in child maltreatment: A meta-analytic review of the literature. Trauma, Violence, & Abuse, 16(4), 471-490. https://doi.org/10.1177/1524838014566728

Standring, S. (2015). Gray's Anatomy: The Anatomical Basis of Clinical Practice (41st ed.). Elsevier Health Sciences.

Sustain Health Magazine. (n.d.). A doctor reveals the link between your mental health and gut health. https://sustainhealth.fit/lifestyle/gut-brain-axis/

Swaab, D. F. (2011). The human hypothalamus in relation to hormonal regulation, emotional and cognitive functioning. Nature Reviews Neuroscience, 12(8), 1-15. https://doi.org/10.1038/nrn3071

The Fulfilled Fork. (n.d.). 5 vagus nerve exercises for better digestion. The Fulfilled Fork. https://thefulfilledfork.com/5-vagus-nerve-exercises-digestion/

The Improvement Artist. (n.d.). Mastering mental grit: Transforming challenges into triumphs. https://www.theimprovementartist.com/mastering-mental-grit-transforming-challenges-into-triumphs/

The Origin Way. (n.d.). Vagus nerve stimulation: 5 techniques that really work. The Origin Way. https://www.theoriginway.com/blog/vagus-nerve-stimulation-5-techniques-that-really-work

Thayer, J. F., & Lane, R. D. (2007). The role of the vagus nerve in the neuroimmune network. Physiology & Behavior, 92(1-2), 67-70. https://doi.org/10.1016/j.pop.2007.05.003

Thayer, J. F., & Lane, R. D. (2012). A model of neurovisceral integration in emotion regulation and dysregulation. Nature Reviews Endocrinology, 8(4), 190-200. https://doi.org/10.1038/nrendo.2012.189

Thayer, J. F., Åhs, F., Fredrikson, M., Sollers, J. J., & Wager, T. D. (2012). A meta-analysis of heart rate variability and neuroimaging studies: Implications for heart rate variability as a marker of stress and health. Brain Imaging and Behavior, 6(3), 256-259. https://doi.org/10.1007/s40473-014-0010-5

Thayer, J. F., Yamamoto, S. S., & Brosschot, J. F. (2018). The relationship of autonomic imbalance, heart rate variability and cardiovascular disease risk factors. Frontiers in Psychiatry, 9, 44. https://doi.org/10.3389/fpsyt.2018.00044

The Shores Recovery. (2021). Vagus nerve stimulation and opioid withdrawal. The Shores Recovery. Retrieved from https://theshoresrecovery.com/vagus-nerve-stimulation-and-opioid-withdrawal/

Tomblin, J. B., & Zhang, X. (2006). The dimensionality of language ability in school-age children. Journal of Speech, Language, and Hearing Research, 49(6), 1193-1208. https://doi.org/10.1044/1092-4388(2008/018)

Tsien, R. W., & Tsien, R. Y. (1998). Calcium channels, stores, and oscillations. Nature, 375(6531), 645-647. https://doi.org/10.1038/35013070

Van der Kolk, B. A. (2014). The Body Keeps the Score: Brain, Mind, and Body in the Healing of Trauma. Viking.

Vibrant Health. (n.d.). Chiropractic. https://www.vibranthealthswfl.com/copy-of-functional-medicine

Vogele, C., & Steptoe, A. (2006). Cardiovascular and metabolic responses to mental stress. Biological Psychology, 72(2), 253-264. https://doi.org/10.1016/j.biopsycho.2006.06.009

Wong, A., Farrand, M. C., Andresen, C., & Beaumont, E. (2021). Vagus nerve stimulation activates nucleus of solitary tract neurons via supramedullary pathways. Journal of Physiology, 599(23), 5261–5279. https://doi.org/10.1113/JP281605

Wu, J. C. (2015). Vagovagal reflex circuits and functions: From the bench to bedside. Neurogastroenterology and Motility, 27(2), 99-112. https://www.ncbi.nlm.nih.gov/pmc/articles/PMC4367209/

Zanos, S., & Tracey, K. J. (2021). Vagus nerve stimulation: Potential benefits and implications for brain health. European Journal of Medical Research, 26, 96. https://doi.org/10.1186/s40001-021-00482-y

Zhou, W., & Pu, Y. (2016). The impact of mindfulness-based stress reduction on well-being and mental health. Neurotherapeutics, 13(2), 372-380. https://doi.org/10.1007/s13311-016-0427-x

Ziegler, M. G., Milic, M., & Sun, P. (2005). Antioxidants, mitochondrial DNA repair, and neuroprotection in Parkinson's disease. Journal of Clinical Investigation, 115(6), 1595-1601. https://doi.org/10.1172/JCI30555

Zipes, D. P., & Rubart, M. (2011). Neural modulation of cardiac arrhythmias and sudden cardiac death. Cardiac Electrophysiology Clinics, 3(1), 35-42. https://doi.org/10.1016/j.ccep.2011.02.009

Made in the USA
Middletown, DE
25 April 2025